# A FRAGILE CIRCLE

## A MEMOIR BY MARK SENAK

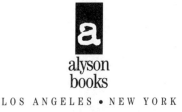

alyson
books

LOS ANGELES • NEW YORK

MANUFACTURED IN THE UNITED STATES OF AMERICA.
PRINTED ON ACID-FREE PAPER.

THIS TRADE PAPERBACK ORIGINAL IS PUBLISHED BY ALYSON PUBLICATIONS INC.,
P.O. BOX 4371, LOS ANGELES, CALIFORNIA 90078-4371.
DISTRIBUTION IN THE UNITED KINGDOM BY TURNAROUND PUBLISHER SERVICES LTD.,
UNIT 3 OLYMPIA TRADING ESTATE, COBURG ROAD, WOOD GREEN,
LONDON N22 6TZ ENGLAND.

FIRST EDITION: JUNE 1998

02 01 00 99 98    10 9 8 7 6 5 4 3 2 1

ISBN 1-55583-460-4


LIBRARY OF CONGRESS CATALOGING-IN-PUBLICATION DATA
    SENAK, MARK S.
        A FRAGILE CIRCLE : A MEMOIR / MARK SENAK.—1ST ED.
        1. SENAK, MARK S.—FRIENDS AND ASSOCIATES. 2. AIDS ACTIVISTS—
    CALIFORNIA—LOS ANGELES—BIOGRAPHY. 3. GAY MEN—CALIFORNIA—
    LOS ANGELES—BIOGRAPHY. I. TITLE
    RC607.A26S432 1998
    362.1'969792'0092—DC21                    98-14570 CIP
    [B]


COVER DESIGN BY CHRISTOPHER HARRITY.
COVER PHOTOGRAPH BY OLIVIER FERRAND.
AUTHOR PHOTOGRAPH BY JANET BELLER.

This book is dedicated
with love to my friends
Michael Lombardo
and
Steven Bing

# CONTENTS

# FOREWORD

I am a fortunate person. I come from a background that has been privileged, and I come from a wonderful family that has used that privilege in the pursuit of philanthropy. And they have been extremely expressive of their compassion in the face of the AIDS epidemic. My mother, Joan Tisch, has served on the board of directors of Gay Men's Health Crisis in New York since 1989. I did my turn with AIDS Project Los Angeles, where I chaired the board of directors for three years. These experiences have demonstrated for me the true meaning of "family values."

Working in AIDS services has been more than largesse on our part. The fight for civil rights and the struggle for basic dignity that we were witness to in our work has reminded me of the heroism of the movement. The battles that have been fought and the courage shown are of epic proportions. It has been a struggle about people who have said they've had enough. Enough of systems that don't work. Enough of doctors who don't treat. Enough of a society that has sometimes let prejudice and fear get in the way of compassion. It has been a story about people who were going to take control over their lives while they have a vision of a better day and find the strength deep from within to fight back.

Because when the history of this epidemic is written, all who have been touched by it will remember it as a war. And like any war, we will mourn those we have lost and cherish our survivors and praise our heroes. The war has been shockingly long—the losses have been unthinkable. Our lovers, our friends, our families and our coworkers—all people lost far too early from our lives. Their unrealized gifts that could have been given to the world, unfulfilled.

It has been a difficult war to wage because we have had to fight it on so many fronts. We are fighting a relentless virus at the same time we have had to fight ignorance, homophobia, and at times our own government. We've even had to fight ourselves because there have been times when we've all just wanted to look away—times when it has been more than we can bear.

The circumstances of the epidemic have changed many times over the years. There has been a promise of hope for the first time with new treatments that for many will add years and quality to their lives. But by no means is the AIDS epidemic over, in fact, because treatments are so expensive and there is so much infection with people who are poor; in some ways the epidemic has merely shifted gears. I fear that if something is not done, we will see new fronts in this war open up and challenge our will and endurance once again.

Still, as we face the future it is important to take stock of where we have been. In *The New York Times Book Review* on March 5, 1995, Patricia Hampl begins a review of a new edition of Anne Frank's diary by quoting the education minister of the Dutch government in exile. On March 28, 1944, he stated that "history cannot be written on the basis of official decisions and documents alone. If your descendants are to understand fully what we as a nation have had to endure and overcome during these years, then what we really need are ordinary documents—

a diary, letters." To this end, he urged his fellow citizens to begin to amass "vast quantities of simple, everyday material."

The principle for which Anne Frank wrote is unchanged. We must record for others exactly what it was like to live through one of the most extraordinary events in the second half of the 20th century—the AIDS epidemic. No other natural disaster will claim so many lives. It is a silent war in our midst, and we live in danger of letting it pass into the oblivion of every other social ill we experience until it is no more a commodity than cancer, homelessness, or drug abuse—problems that have become so big that we feel we cannot overcome them; so on some level we accept them.

The thoughts and feelings of the early days of the epidemic stand in danger of being forgotten or having never been recorded at all. Events are there for posterity, recorded in our newspapers and in books such as *And the Band Played On*. But such sources do not on their own tell the story, especially since they are written from the journalistic perspective rather than the insider's. What would our perception of the Vietnam War be if we merely relied on newspaper and journalists' accounts of what happened?

There aren't many witnesses left. Mark Senak joined 17 other staff members at Gay Men's Health Crisis, having first volunteered in 1982 and later in 1985 became employed there. GMHC is the oldest and largest AIDS service organization in the world. Of those 18 people, only six are known to the author to be alive; only four are gay men. The number of people who can write this book are fewer and fewer in number. Mark Senak has written us a long letter home from the front lines of the silent war of the AIDS epidemic.

We will find strength, I believe, in our future challenges by looking to the heroism of the past. In the face of idle promises and indifference, an entire culture of people rose up to care for themselves—when no one else was going to do it—by creating AIDS service organizations and becoming more activist about their disease than anything seen before. This community of caring people did this despite their own fatigue and overwhelming sadness, and it is their courage and their anger that motivate us. And it is their hearts and their ability in the face of this hell that have inspired compassion in others. Heroes are called upon to do more than they think themselves capable of, and it is that extra measure of giving—when you have nothing left to give—that has made heroes out of ordinary people throughout the epidemic.

Sometimes the HIV/AIDS experience has been defined by statistics. Unfortunately, we've gotten so good at quantifying AIDS that we can tell you how many people are infected each day, how many people die each hour, and how many people we've lost by age, region, and country of origin. *A Fragile Circle* defines it differently. Behind every statistic is a human being: a friend, a lover, a father, a brother, a son. Each with a history, a heart, a face, and a soul. They are the people described in this book.

Each person touched by the epidemic has had an intensely personal struggle. Some struggles make it to court and the newspapers. Most are quiet battles—fights with insurance companies to keep coverage and use benefits, fights with government agencies to qualify for and receive benefits, fights with health care agencies to get quality care in a timely manner. Some are even more basic fights for food and shelter. Some are the fights one faces when you have to carry on knowing you've lost the most important person in your world.

Each of us needs to commit and indeed recommit ourselves to taking steps every day. We can't count on others to take responsibility; it has to come from within, as Mark Senak so poignantly points out to us in this book. For indeed the only way we can combat this inhumane epidemic is by mustering every bit of humanity we have and remembering our long and proud tradition of compassion and service.

Steve Tisch
Los Angeles
March 1998

# ACKNOWLEDGMENTS

Everyone who put up with me during the writing of this book deserves a bigger thank you than I can extend to them in these words. Wherever and whoever you are, thank you.

But there are people who stand out. My friend Michael Lombardo encouraged me throughout this project to keep writing it and understood completely when I called him late at night just to blather about it. My friend Kate Graber held up her end by doing the same; with a steadfast loyalty she reminded me every time I got down about it that she loved me, which was a very important encouragement.

I have had the good fortune to have in my boss at the time, Jimmy Loyce, a person who combines the unique skills of a clinician with those of a friend. He is the truest human being I have ever worked for, and his encouragement and support have been more appreciated than I will ever get to say to him. I love him very much for that and more and for judiciously applying several coats of confidence to my thin veneer of ego. Poor Jimmy could have written this book himself, because I told him all these stories more than once over many lunches. He is a hero to me and to the entire movement of people who work in AIDS.

Dan Bross and Bob Cundall offered me both hospitality and encouragement, and Dan was a reader of the manuscript in its early form, and for that they are both owed thanks, especially since large portions of this was written in their Virginia home.

Christine Lubinski was also a reader, and I am grateful for her suggestions. Early encouragement also came from Jane Rosette.

John D'Amico was a reader whose insights provided me with perspective when I could get none. I have had the good fortune to be blessed with many friends, several of whom took the time to also read and comment on the book, including Bill Jones and RoMa Johnson. My thanks also to Hope Tshopik-Schneider for many good conversations and elegant lunches during the writing of this book.

John Gile and Victoria Sharp helped me finish this book by taking me skiing, and for that, among other things, I am most grateful.

All the best intentions would be for nothing were it not for the professional side of the equation. My agent, Laurie Harper, was determined to sell this manuscript, and her tenacity for doing just that outweighed my own. As down as I could get, which can be pretty down, she would balance with up.

Gerry Kroll also exhibited a faith and enthusiasm for this project that surprised and touched me, and I am very obliged to him for both his sentiment and his commitment to this work. Kevin Bentley was a very skilled editor, and his talent made this a far better work than it was. My thanks also to my publisher, Greg Constante, who consistently expressed his faith in this project, which meant a lot. My gratitude also goes to David Epstein and Ann Moravick, who, for different reasons, have helped me out with a new lease on life.

Lastly, my family needs to be thanked, because within these pages there is much of them and the values taught to me by my mother and my sister.

# INTRODUCTION

## *Dodgeball*

During my freshman year in high school, a time I remember to be fraught with hormones and uncertainty, I, like so many of my yet-to-be gay colleagues, dreaded that period of the school day known as physical education. The irony of this, of course, is that while we shunned it then, today we pay considerable sums of money each year to belong to affluent gyms where we pump up our bodies, overcompensating for our aversions back then.

There is an incident in my PE class that often comes back to me these days. It is not the memory of being afraid to undress in front of the other boys or of being swatted with a wooden paddle by a coach for not wearing a jock strap (yes, they actually did that to us and, yes, it was in a public, not private or religious, school), nor is it a memory of forging some kind of doctor's note as a way to get out of gym, although that would not have been beneath me.

This specific day was in winter. On rainy winter days the coaches couldn't think of anything for us to do but to play a game called dodgeball. The object of this game, as most of us remember, is for two teams to separate on both sides of the gymnasium and begin throwing large rubber balls at one another. The coaches, long past their prime, would sit on the sidelines, blowing their whistles like judges at a dance contest when a member of one team would cause a member of the opposing team to be "out." This was accomplished by hitting an opponent with the ball and sending him out of the game to the purgatory of the sidelines. If a member of the opposing team could catch the ball hurled at him, then the thrower was out. For this, the coaches had gone to college.

I used to pray to get "out" quickly, which was not an easy task, for throwing a ball too gently so that it would be caught by the opposite team was a dead giveaway that you were a "soft sissy." Even though I knew who I was at the not-so-tender age of 13, I was hardly ready to broadcast it in my junior high school. On the other hand, throwing the ball in a real effort to try and get someone on the other team "out" ran the substantial risk of incurring that person's wrath for the next game. Getting hit by a ball often caused a bruise that didn't go away for days. Getting hit square in the face is something I don't even want to recall, but I remember watching it happen to someone else with the same fascination with which one would witness a car wreck.

Somehow, on this particular day, through the agonizing process of elimination, I found myself left alone on my team. Solo—facing off with just one team member on the opposing side. Until the United States invaded Granada, there would never be a more pathetic match.

I stood on my half of the gym, a poorly defended territory, my teammates screaming at the sidelines. The flaccid rubber balls gathered around like pigeons on pavement, while on the other side of the gym stood Jon. Jon was not a school athlete; he was *the* school athlete. He *looked forward* to PE. He probably even looked forward to dodgeball.

Jon was muscular, and his facial expression was set in an adult fashion that rarely changed, lending an air of control and toughness. He was on every team—baseball and football—and when people looked at him, even teachers, they were a little bit afraid. He wasn't your clean-cut athlete; he was the type of boy who, commanding the strength of a man, had a certain knowing sophistication that probably would not stick with him throughout his life. This is best expressed by the fact that he smoked, which in those days was sophisticated. He even inhaled. He looked older than my dad.

Jon, his arms girded with a musculature simply unnatural in one so young, was thrusting rubber balls at me with a velocity that caused them to make very loud noises, hurting my ears when I dodged them. There was no one I could hide behind. My highest hope was to get out of the game without getting hit in the face.

Shouts came from all around and echoed up to the girders near the ceiling like frightened bats in a cave. The gym transformed itself into the Coliseum, and these boys either wanted to see blood or wanted to win, shouting out for their preference as if their very lives depended on it. It is the thing I remember the most. Left alone facing my powerful adversary, I would have gladly traded places with any of them.

I was a runner. I had good legs, and they served me well while I dutifully dodged Jon's throws. It kept my face intact and was lending a high sense of drama to the contest. Having survived his numerous attacks, I kept trying to pick up the balls and throw them back at him, but he threw them at me with such force they usually bounced right back to him before I could pick one up. If by chance I did get hold of a ball and throw it, it never made the sound his did. Sometimes they didn't even reach the opposite wall. I usually threw so wide that he couldn't catch them because they didn't come anywhere near him. I began to lose my breath, and while I gasped for air I thought I could see a glimmer of faint amusement in the blue eyes set so deeply in that otherwise stoic face.

And then, like the hare with the tortoise, he made his mistake. He turned his back. He turned his back on me to pick up a ball resting at the back of his side of the gym. It was a thoughtless and arrogant mistake. I spotted the only ball on my side of the court, lying there like debris from a bombing. I tossed it in the air in his direction. It rose in a long and graceful arc, and the crowd of boys began to scream a warning to him that it was coming, but he didn't catch on. With his back to me and reaching for another ball to lob my way, my missile glanced off his shoulder—and he was out.

The next thing I knew, all my teammates came rushing out to me, screaming as they picked me up. I remember that I could barely breathe from exhaustion, though I was still able to note that odor peculiar to sweaty adolescent boys. My lungs hurt. The exhilaration of the crowd of boys seemed almost animal and though I tried to share in their thrill and disbelief, I could feel only pain, fatigue, and a vague perception of relief that I had somehow escaped harm.

We are now well into the 17th year of the HIV health crisis. When I began working at the Gay Men's Health Crisis in 1985, there were 18 employees. Of those 18 people, I believe that only six of us are still alive. It is a most peculiar feeling not to even be able to remember everyone's name, just like the boys on my team that day. The people I worked with, the people I dated, people who were friends. I cannot always remember their names. Some of the time I cannot even remember what they looked like. They stand on the sidelines where I can't see them.

Then there are friends I do remember. The people who came to my house for dinners, the people I dated, the people I loved: Joe, Neil, Carter, Mitchell, Allen, Lou, Paul, Rick (the funniest man on earth and now the funniest in heaven), Brad, Grif, Michael, another Michael, and yet another Michael, and Richard…and so many others.

I try to think about what all of this means. Every so often I see another one of my friends depart. I worry that the next one might be me. I worry that I'll catch it right in the face and that my "out" won't be easy. I don't know any more if I'll make it to the end of the game; I don't know if I want to be the last one left. Longevity is no longer my goal. Longevity is lonely and it hurts, and afterward I'm not sure that I'll be left with anything other than the vague perception that I have escaped some unspeakable harm, like that day so long ago.

Every 15 seconds someone in the world is infected with HIV. It is a good thing I cannot make friends that fast.

There is no end in sight, despite the dramatic developments with protease inhibitors that have made such a difference in the quality of life for people with HIV. Even if a cure could be found, with HIV having infected at least 17 million people worldwide—an estimated 40 million to be infected over the next five years (mostly in Africa and Asia)— a cure will most likely have to be oral and cheap; neither seems likely right now.

And from the sidelines I can hear the faint echo of the shouts and murmurs of all my dead friends and colleagues, and I wait for the chance when just for one damned moment my opponent turns his back. Then the sound of my teammates will no longer be faint; they'll rush up to me from the sidelines, screaming and shouting and picking me up because at last the game will be over and we will have won.

Mark Senak
Los Angeles
January 1998

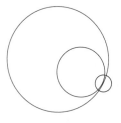

# PART ONE

## UNKNOWN SOLDIERS

*"I was afraid of a dog,*
*until I saw a lion."*

**~THE TALMUD~**

CHAPTER 1 : 1 9 8 1

---

*301 cases of AIDS were diagnosed*
*120 people died*
*A cumulative total of 389 cases were diagnosed*
*150 people were dead of AIDS in America*

---

## PROVIDENCE OR ACCIDENT?

When it all began a lot of people asked me how and why I got into AIDS work. Sometimes now, people still do ask. I often ask this of myself. This line of questioning starts me thinking about the roles of Providence and Accident in my life. Unsure what it is that guides us through the space and time we live in, there are times when I begin my day wondering whether my day, my existence, my purpose was the product of some plan or just some series of random accidents. The multitude of possibilities that exist from one moment to the next spawn a flurry of "ifs" and "what ifs," crowding my consciousness like commuters on a subway train. They swirl and punch, in a hurry to get to wherever it is that they are going, to accomplish whatever it is they need to accomplish, and then to come back the next day and do it all over again. What happened today maybe wouldn't have happened at all if I had turned left instead of right or taken a different route to the store or stayed at work a few minutes longer or went to a movie instead of doing the laundry. From the most mundane decisions come monumental consequences in our lives.

I thought a lot about the role of Providence and Accident even before AIDS. Then, when the epidemic began, I spent countless hours wondering about people I saw as clients and the series of events that led up to this moment, to the destruction of their lives, to having me sitting there next to them doing their deathbed will. What twist of fate, what series of accidents brought us both to that room at that time? I was afforded these countless hours of ponderings on New York City subways, going to and coming home from appointments with dying people. They haunted my dreams.

But then when AIDS began to really hit, and hit hard, by the end of the day, none of this mattered anymore. When people I knew began dying more quickly than I could have imagined and when I found myself too burned-out to go to the memorial services of my friends and colleagues, my philosophizing slowed to a crawl. When my address book, like so many other people's, became less a resource than a painful reminder of friends who no longer existed, my meanderings stopped completely. I was no longer an interested observer who was helping out; I was suddenly in the center of risk, waiting and wondering whether or not I would live. For me, in the early days of this epidemic I no longer had the luxury to ponder, but rather each day was a bit like being in a car wreck. It was less important to know how it happened than it was to know that you were all right.

My friend John D'Amico says that in those early days we thought the world was flat, but now we know it is round. The place where I live now is a place where we know many of the ins and outs of HIV and AIDS and of life and death. But the memories that are the bulk of my life all occurred when the world was flat, and they are echoes of a time and mentality that doesn't exist anymore.

## JUST LIKE THE CLAP

There was a man in my life named Todd who has the distinction of being the first person I dated over a period of time, making it a "relationship." One Saturday morning we were lying in bed still in disarray from a bout of morning passion, a passion which had not been "safe" by today's standards. Todd, who was reading a newspaper, told me about a new disease that was being called GRID, which stood for gay related immune deficiency. I hadn't heard much about it, but as he read the description to me from the local gay rag, I really did have that horrible sense of cold fingers trying to grab onto my beating heart. That is not to say my response was prophetic; I am always subject to panicky feelings around issues of health. But this was more than passing paranoia—it was my instinct. I wanted him to stop reading, but I didn't say anything. He said people were dying from this new disease quickly and that mostly homosexuals were getting it. As soon as he said it, my mind worked itself into a state I like to call the Maginot Line of Logic. I imagine the worst-case scenario, prepare like hell for it, and find that my enemy can usually just walk around it.

Weeks later Todd and I were drinking our morning coffee as he read yet another article out loud to me. The reason Todd was so often reading these articles to me was that I refused to read them myself. It was something I would rather avoid. When it came to matters of health, I was a gay version of Woody Allen. If I read about it, I knew I would have it. If I knew the symptoms, I would begin to imagine and even experience them. On the other hand, ignorance being bliss, if I didn't know about it, I reasoned, then I wouldn't get too afraid. This, I later learned, was a process called denial, and we would all become familiar with it as the epidemic unfolded.

Todd put the paper down. "Oh well," he shrugged, "in a few years, it'll be like the clap. You'll get a shot, and that'll be the end of it." He looked smug and comfortable, as if to say, "Our science can beat up your germ."

This took me a moment to comprehend. I had never had the clap. The benefit of having several health neuroses is that sexually, I had always been conservative and always been careful. What I mean by that is that I didn't just jump into bed with anyone I'd met and exchange bodily fluids. Intimacy was important to me and, as luck would have it, Todd was the first person with whom I'd felt that intimacy. Up until 1981 I'd been sexual with only people in ways that were deemed "safe" after the epidemic started. But being in a relationship, I had finally thrown out any inhibitions with Todd. I looked at him now as he spoke with a chill. He had more than once referred to his past of going to the "tubs," and it didn't take great leaps of logic to suspect that Todd had not been so careful and that the voice with which he spoke about the clap was one of experience.

I shook my head. "No, Todd, I think it sounds more complicated than that," I said. In most arguments that I had ever had with Todd, I was usually right. In this one I would have liked to have been wrong.

Years later in 1987 I would hear about a study done to see what caused some people to stay in AIDS work longer than others. One of the things that came to light was the expectation people had of the epidemic when it began. Those who thought it would be short-lived, burned out when it turned out to be long-lived. Those who thought it would last for a long time, tended to last longer doing AIDS work. I was surprised at the results of the study—not because the result was necessarily so unexpected but because so many people had originally thought that the epidemic wouldn't last. Granted, Todd had not thought that it would last, but even at the zenith of our relationship I had never thought that Todd had the sense God gave a can of paint. The year before, Todd and I were in Vermont at the weekend home of my friends Anna and Tom for a little skiing. It was near dusk and the house, located on a remote 350-acre tract, stood in the midst of a long, gently sloping meadow. I was unpacking our suitcases while Todd stood looking out the window at the serenity of the freshly snow-filled meadow as it reflected the fading light.

"Look," said Todd. "Sheep!"

"Sheep?" I asked. This was somewhat surprising. I had been coming to this spot in Vermont for quite a long time, and I had never seen any sheep in the area. I knew that Tom and Anna's friends had never kept any livestock and was concerned that someone might be using the property without permission to store sheep. Since they were not with us, I would have to act as caretaker and ward off some sheep farmer. I went to the window and put my arm around Todd's shoulders and peered outside. "Where?"

"There. Right there." Todd pointed to silhouetted forms walking in formation in the distance. I peered at them.

"Todd," I said patiently, "those are wild turkeys. Sheep have four legs. Turkeys have only two." Laughing at him, I added, "Sheep, Todd, do not fly, and generally they do not have feathers." In short, relying on Todd's good sense would indeed be taking a big risk. But relying on him was just what I was doing. Later that winter night in 1981 we had sex that today we know was very unsafe.

To his credit, Todd did make me discuss GRID with him. We began to talk about it a lot. At times I felt like putting my hands over my ears and singing loudly so that I couldn't hear him.

This was all before there was any such thing as the concept of "safe sex." At first, that is what they called it—"safe sex". Later, when it proved that the only safe sex was no sex, it was changed to "safer sex". But it seemed clear that the more conservative one was, the safer one was. Safe, to me, meant not having other partners but remaining within a relationship.

Later Todd assured me that I could feel safe from the "gay plague" as he and others came to call it; it was a term that made me inwardly wince. He claimed that doctors were saying that the reason some gay men were dying was because they had done too many drugs and had experienced several bouts of venereal diseases. The antibiotics, the frequent exposures, the drugs, and the late hours, they theorized, had combined forces like some moral legion organized to punish and wear down the immune system of people in the fast lane. Ironically, there are some people today who still subscribe wholeheartedly to this theory. These are people who, I think, are too afraid to take the time to understand the epidemic. I was the same way back then in 1981, when I didn't want to read any articles or to acknowledge this new disease in any real way. It made it easier for me then, and I guess it makes it easier today for people who still don't know someone with AIDS.

But this theory of AIDS was great for me. I liked it. It had so much of a moral element to it. And I knew it wouldn't affect me because I was very, very moral. It was just what I had been looking for to make me feel safe from the "dreaded disease," as news people liked to call it when they bothered to talk about it at all.

In a recently conducted poll about sexually transmitted diseases, most Americans said that they would never acquire a sexually transmitted disease, yet it is estimated that one in four do. I am happy to say I did not invent denial.

Then, no one talked publicly about an infectious agent causing the syndrome, and science was far from discovering a virus. But at some point not long after he introduced it to me, I began to doubt Todd's report of the developing promiscuity theory in the back of my mind. Flaws in the logic began to appear almost immediately like threads in a cheap suit. After all, I lived in New York City, where homosexuals most certainly did not corner the market on drugs and sex. I also knew Haitians, one of the other "high-risk groups," weren't leading lifestyles similar to gay men. Common sense, if not empirical science, said that it must be something infectious. It seems obvious now, but then there was something of a quality of science fiction to the idea that there was a new disease. After all, how often did new diseases suddenly crop up out of nowhere?

No, insisted Todd. It was only those leather queens who stayed out all night licking the streets who were getting it, he said. It would be their problem, not ours. While I privately rolled my eyes at his naïveté, I nevertheless allowed myself to feel relieved, and Todd and I clung to this theory like a life raft while we continued to play Russian roulette with our bodies and our lives.

Since the beginning of the epidemic, everyone has at some point grabbed onto this life raft of belief—of needing to believe that AIDS is somebody else's problem. It is a pattern that has echoed down the history of the epidemic. No one wants to believe that he or she is at risk, preferring to believe that the death and destruction are someone else's problem. And whosever problem it is, should by all means be blamed. Moral reprehension has historically accompanied the act of getting sick in America. I knew better back then. But in 1981 engaging in denial by saying that it was someone else's problem seemed like the safest thing to do.

# CHAPTER 2 : 1982

---

*1,143 new cases of AIDS were diagnosed*
*446 more people died*
*A cumulative total of 1,532 cases were diagnosed*
*596 people were dead of AIDS in America*

---

## SOMEONE DIES

During the period of January to June 1982, 151 people died of AIDS-related complications in the United States. The first person I knew who died of AIDS was one of those people. He managed to die of the disease before it had a real name. His name was Jeff, and I met him at a large Wall Street law firm, where he was a lawyer and I was a student working my way through law school during the late 1970s as a legal secretary and word processor. He was young and successful and had a pleasant attitude, particularly when you compared him with most other lawyers at big Wall Street firms.

I was intrigued by him because he was about the only gay lawyer in the firm who didn't go out of his way to hide the fact, though there were certainly others. Being gay then was safer than it had been, but it still wasn't something about which people were terribly open. I had only just come out of college and had not really had the experience of meeting many people who felt they could be openly gay, much less in a large and professional atmosphere.

When I began law school in 1978 I worked at the firm on a part-time basis. One day Jeff called me to interrogate me about my law school, Brooklyn Law School in Brooklyn Heights, because it turned out he was considering going to teach there. It was a logical move because although the firm was open-minded enough to tolerate a gay associate, it was probably not in the market for a gay partner. There were partners who were rumored to be gay, but if they were, they were men who managed to keep their secret until after they had achieved their higher, tenured status, and even then they maintained the title of "bachelor." Jeff began to teach at the law school in 1981 and became my coach for moot-court competitions, which are contests involving mock trials.

One evening while I was walking down Christopher Street in Greenwich Village, I crossed paths with Jeff. I almost didn't recognize him. He was wearing a leather vest and a small leather cap, tame by today's standards. I was amused and scandalized at the same time. I think I had some preconceived notions about people who might be active on the sexual scene and particularly people who might wear leather that wasn't part of their shoes, watchband or sensible belt—and my notions had told me that they weren't people like Jeff. But he was nice, and I always liked him, so my stereotype was challenged, given that he wore Brooks Brothers button-down shirts, corduroys, and a lightweight spring London Fog jacket as he coached me through court competitions.

Then in 1982, the year after I graduated, he took a leave of absence from teaching at the school and never came back. He died, I think, in the spring of that year, and I went to his memorial service, held in the same moot-court room in which he had coached me.

At Jeff's memorial Todd's words about who was getting this disease and why echoed in my head. I remembered seeing Jeff in his leather vest. Who knew? Maybe Todd was right.

It was not Jeff's death that served as a springboard to launch me into a career in AIDS work, but all the same, later in the following year I was doing deathbed wills for people dying of AIDS even though the merest thought of it chilled me. The hows and whys of it still lead me to the inevitable cycle of pondering over Providence and Accident.

## I GRAB A CAB, THE DOORS ARE OPEN

Any New Yorker will, upon being asked, admit that there is a certain art to hailing a cab. It is an artform enhanced by the occasion of rain. It is not the simple matter of stepping out from the curb and putting up a yearning hand in signal to some available hack that you want a ride. It's more complicated than that. It requires a great deal of mental thought, energy, and sometimes endurance. Your thought waves have to be heavier than those of your opponents. And it is only the most consummate New Yorker who can do this without it appearing as though he or she is really trying. Tourists don't stand a chance. But it is truly a mark of distinction when a cab stops to pick you up before you have raised your hand, or in my case, before I even stepped off the curb. But that is exactly how I got introduced to the notion of working with people with AIDS.

During law school I lived in the Park Slope section of Brooklyn. Park Slope is a collection of old brownstones located on a gentle hill coming down from Prospect Park. The house I lived in reportedly was once owned by Al Smith, the presidential candidate who lost to Herbert Hoover in 1928. In 1982 the neighborhood was an odd mix of ethnicities and young urban professionals who were busy gentrifying the area.

Coming home from work on the subway one evening, I had noticed an exceptionally tall, slender man who had nice eyes and great skin tone. He got off the subway at the same stop I did on the F train in from Manhattan. I could always spot him in the neighborhood shopping because he was so extremely tall. The fact that he was extremely thin also made him appear even taller. I did not know his name, and we never really spoke except to say hello, but I could always spot him from far away—even among other tall, thin men—because he had what my father called taxicab ears, a reference to a view of a taxicab from the front with doors open on both sides. He had large ears that stood out from his head a bit, and I found this unusual effect very attractive. He lived one street over from me. I began to take walks around the block in the hope that I would run into him, and sometimes I was lucky. Then we would stop to talk at the fence that surrounded the small courtyard in front of his brownstone, and my hunch about him was correct; he was intelligent. Intelligent, interesting men are in my book hard to find. Many times if you're lucky enough to find one who is intelligent, he's a boor. The worst is when he is a boor and not intelligent. So in fact it has been my experience that "intelligent, interesting men" is a phrase that is an oxymoron. But this guy was truly both.

One day during the thrill of a curbside conversation with my tall neighbor, he told me he was going to be moving away from New York to attend law school in the South, which as it turned out was back home for him. I was miffed. It had taken me weeks just to get the nerve up to begin having these brief conversations with him in the neighborhood, and now he was just up and moving away. Having just finished and taken the bar exam, I tried to talk him out of this law-school folly, but he said he was sure that it was what he wanted to do. As a mere neighbor, it turned out I didn't have much sway in his life plans. He moved away, and the neighborhood became a little less interesting. I got a job at an investment firm. Not long afterward I moved into Manhattan, back to the upper west side, where I had first lived when I arrived in New York as a 21-year-old college graduate with a not-too-marketable degree in creative writing.

Several months later while at the east end of Jones Beach, the gay section, I spotted someone who caught my attention. I was alone and it was hot and the beach was as usual fairly crowded. I had been sitting there reading a trash novel and soaking up the sun's rays to ensure that I would prematurely age and later on have skin cancer to worry about when I saw an unmistakable tall, thin silhouette several yards away. Only a glance at the taxicab door ears was necessary for me to know that the guy down the beach was the guy who had lived around the corner from me. I hadn't even known his name. I got up and ran over to him to say hello and ask how law school was.

He told me that he had dropped out. In exchange I wore my smug "I told you so" look. He told me that he had come back to take a job with Gay Men's Health Crisis, the new organization set up to help men who had what was now being called AIDS. He was going to be the new executive director. His name was Rodger McFarlane. The agency, located in the basement of a brownstone in Chelsea, had only a few paid staff. They were doing education and providing a service that became known as the Buddy Program, to have volunteers help guys out who were sick and abandoned by family, friends, and the system. The same thing was beginning to happen in large cities around the country. GMHC's motto, however—First in the fight against AIDS—is true. What started out during a meeting of a few concerned people in Larry Kramer's living room resulted in the first effort in that Chelsea basement. It grew into a $30-million service organization. What it will become next to meet the changing landscape of HIV services is unknown. That day at Jones Beach, Rodger had a genuine excitement in his eyes and his voice as he told me about what he was doing that I would later discover is the way Rodger talks about anything when he is "on." Rodger has a way of making any losing situation sound like a winner. He can make the act of taking out the garbage sound hot and hip and exciting. But the very thought of what he was telling me was very depressing, and made my stomach queasy. I graciously tried to change the subject.

Rodger was what the media had dubbed an "AIDS activist." I was not then and I'm still not today at all sure of what that term is supposed to mean. I think most people immediately visualize guys who throw blood on the carpets of other people, a tactic later sometimes employed by the group ACT UP, the AIDS Coalition to Unleash Power. When I have been interviewed on television news those words—AIDS activist—have frequently appeared under my image. Yet I can't imagine writing it down on my tax return as my occupation. But I knew as Rodger spoke that that's what he was—an AIDS activist.

And as he spoke I mentally distanced myself from the man. To say that I sensed too much danger in what he said to me is an understatement. He simply was going too far. I knew I should run the other way. Other than Jeff, I did not know anyone who had "it." Nor did I want to know anyone. I had just begun to feel safe wrapped up in the armor of Todd's disease theories, and now Rodger was standing there on the beach poking, holes all through it. The very thought of what he was about to do with his life and his career filled me with fear. I was terrified about AIDS, afraid even of my own sexuality. Just talking to an AIDS activist was tough. I wasn't all that comfortable being "out" with my sexual orientation to anyone but my mixed circle of friends, a feeling that was not that uncommon back then. AIDS brought a lot of us out of the closet, sometimes feet first.

I still believed—because I wanted to believe—that only promiscuous men got it. I wanted to believe that I was safe. But just the fact that something like a GMHC was emerging made me grossly uncomfortable, it somehow made AIDS permanent. And the thought of a couple of guys in a brownstone basement trying to buck what was happening was sort of like a gay rights thing. It was grassroots and hopeless. What Rodger described as this organization sounded like that in some way. It was gay sex, gay rights, death and dying, mysterious illness, drugs; it was everything I was afraid of contemplating. As a gay man, I felt tremendous sympathy, but becoming involved in the way

Rodger was doing meant putting myself out there in a way I didn't think I could ever do. I told him that but told him that I really admired what he was going to try to do. What, after all, could they really hope to accomplish? No one would ever give them any money; there was too much stigma.

"I could never do anything like that," I said. He smiled and said, "You never know, honey. Write up a proposal of some kind, and we might do it."

"Right," I thought with a lot of sarcasm, and I went back to my beach towel, haunted and intimidated, as if I had just watched a man go off to war while I stayed home and dodged the draft. My languid and restful read on the beach turned into an afternoon of high anxiety, blossoming neurosis, and the beginning of a long process of examination of my paranoia and hypocrisy.

Rodger served as executive director from 1982 to 1985. During that time the agency grew from a handful of people and a budget of a few thousand dollars to a staff of about 50 with a budget of a few million. Today people sometimes fault Rodger for his political outlook or his affiliation with the vitriolic but altogether necessary Larry Kramer. But it was just such people who could have taken GMHC from a brownstone basement to a world-class operation. Rodger and the people who worked at GMHC with him during that time will always be heroes in my estimation, deserving the unqualified respect of anyone touched by HIV. As a subculture, we are far too self-destructive to allow ourselves anything too close to a hero, but if we ever change our ways, people like Rodger will go into a hall of fame. His innocently laid out challenge to me to "write up a proposal" turned out to be pretty prophetic.

# CHAPTER 3 : 1983

---

*3,021 new cases of AIDS were diagnosed*
*1,470 more people died*
*A cumulative total of 4,553 cases were diagnosed*
*2,066 people were dead of AIDS in America*

---

## MOTHER TERESA IN A FLANNEL SHIRT

It was the winter of 1982–1983 when Mark Hemphill, a friend of mine I had met taking the bar exam, told me that he was going to go to a meeting of some lawyers who had gotten together to volunteer time to write wills for people with AIDS. I decided to go for no other reason than that I liked the person who asked me to go, and thinking of Jeff, I was curious.

The group met in an apartment in my neighborhood on the upper west side of Manhattan. It was snowing that night. I always found New York in snow to be the most charming event, even when it was a devastating snow storm. The great metropolis was humbled by a snowfall like a sinner before a simple cloudlike vision of God, and for a few hours it was hushed and reverent, as though all was right with the world. Life slowed down, and people stopped long enough to think about and perhaps even appreciate the things they otherwise had no time to contemplate. A few days or sometimes only hours later, of course, as the blanket of snow gave way to a sea of slush, which grew like kudzu at every street corners, we would all return to our winters of discontent.

The group of volunteer lawyers worked under the auspices of the Bar Association for Human Rights of Greater New York, a lesbian and gay group. This unwieldy name was born from compromise, brought on by the fact that several of the lawyers—in emotional and blustery speeches couched in a lifetime of fear—stated that they would leave and form their own organization if the words *lesbian* and *gay* were included the group's name. As it turned out, I was not the only one with insecure feelings about being out of the closet, especially on this issue. Even so, I was already making some progress in my own sense of outrage about AIDS and felt compelled that if we were being put upon with this disease, then we should stand up and make ourselves heard without shame because shame, along with the disease, would be one of our most deadly enemies. Thus, I was one of the vocal supporters of putting the words *lesbian* and *gay* into our association's name. Much drama ensued. It was ironic that while people were dying in hospitals, we spent time and anger in great debate over whether we could identify ourselves as gays and lesbians while helping them. In the end we compromised in the interest of getting on to more important things. Before the epidemic got much further along, AIDS would bring us all out, one way or another, screaming and kicking, sometimes at each other, sometimes at government, sometimes against our own mortality. Sooner or later we all stepped across the line. This incident is typical of the kind of trouble people can have when they work together, spending so much time on a seemingly unimportant detail. It isn't confined to the gay community; after all, while men died in Vietnam, negotiators argued in Paris over the shape of the conference table. A visit to one of the Ryan White councils of various cities today will show that this human propensity hasn't gone away over time. So we settled on the Bar Association for Human Rights of Greater New York because it was "code" for *lesbian* and *gay*.

The chairperson of the pro bono panel of the association was the Mother Teresa of all lawyers, a man named Steve Gittleson. He was as unlikely a hero as any man or woman I have ever met, yet the words "sainted hero" apply to him.

In appearance he was sometimes hapless and careless. He was a lawyer who looked comfortable only in flannel shirts and jeans or on special occasions in thick-ribbed corduroys. He had what I call watercolor eyes—big pools of brown—and his expression was always a combination of wonderment and anxiety, eyebrows always arched in inquiring anticipation. Chain-smoking Benson and Hedges and drinking gallons of coffee a day, a cloudburst of nervous energy hung around him forming an almost visible haze. He was the only person I ever saw who could keep a cigarette in his mouth while he drank a cup of coffee. He was always, always drinking coffee. I remember one summer day—one of those really disgusting, garbage-everywhere-smelling days so unique to New York summertime, when the humidity is in a hostile contest with oppressive heat to determine which can be most relentless—Steve and I went out to lunch. It was too hot to really eat, and I could barely tolerate the thought of some cold gazpacho and a frozen margarita. Steve, on the other hand, in a flannel shirt, ordered a cheeseburger and a cup of coffee. That, I think, was the key to his survival and aptitude in this time of crisis; maybe he was just oblivious to it all on some level. No one would know what Steve looked like without his cloud of energy. The characterization of a deer caught in headlights is an overused one, but it is also the most apt in Steve's case. Perhaps he saw all too clearly what was going on. Beginning the work of assembling a lot of frightened lawyers to do work that no one wanted to do was visionary. He made us surprise ourselves as individuals and as a group.

Steve sat in meetings of the pro bono panel with a wooden box of index cards perched on one knee and an ashtray on the other, his coffee cup somewhere in reach. In the box he had index cards on which he had clients' names with the type of cases they presented, such as will preparation, landlord-tenant disputes, insurance-related matters, or incidences of discrimination. In another he had lawyers' names.

He made assignments to those of us volunteering. There were about 15 or 20 faithfuls who regularly showed up at the meetings. Clients' requests for legal assistance were made from the workers at Gay Men's Health Crisis, where my handsome, former Brooklyn neighbor, Rodger McFarlane, was struggling to make the organization viable and accepted. Steve received the cases and assigned them to the volunteers and, accordingly, the volunteers met with the clients and assisted in the legal matter free of charge. The pro bono panel handled wills and powers-of-attorney preparations mostly. Soon, however, other legal problems occurred, and the panel began answering people's needs in the landlord-tenant disputes and in discrimination cases. Later it would take on debtor-creditor problems and insurance-related issues.

Some of the lawyers who did this work were social misfits, some were sophisticated; all were devoted, loyal, and wonderful people who had a clear commitment to helping people who had real need and who in 1983 were friendless. Now knowing that some of those lawyers have died themselves, I know that there are that many less generous and heroic people in the world. I know that there are less than there should be.

## THEORY BECOMES PRACTICE

People who had AIDS died very quickly in those days. Until 1985 there was no HIV antibody test. There was no known virus causing the disease. Transmission routes seemed uncertain, although doctors were saying very early on that it was spread by sexual contact and bodily fluids, not by casual transmission. In those days people found out they were infected when they first contracted an opportunistic infection, which would take advantage of the body's weakened immune system. In fact, it became apparent that AIDS doesn't cause one to get new illnesses. Rather, you become more susceptible to any virus and bacteria that you already harbor in your system, which makes you ill once you no longer have an immune system to protect you. So out of the blue, a person feeling relatively well one day would suddenly have cancer or pneumocystis pneumonia. Doctors were not skilled in treating these opportunistic infections, and people died within a matter of months from the time of their first illness. With much of the first wave of diagnoses among white gay men, one of the most pressing need many clients presented was for a last will and testament.

Wills class was one of the classes in law school that I aced. Up until this point the type of law I was practicing was corporate at the investment firm. My first pro bono AIDS legal case was for a man who was a vice president of a major publishing house. He was going to come to my home for an initial will interview. Afterward, I would draw up a draft and send it to him and he would edit and return it. Then we would draw up a final copy, and I would supervise the execution of the will.

He was to arrive early on a Saturday afternoon. When the day came I was a nervous wreck. I had never knowingly met a person with AIDS before, and I had never written a will. I cannot even remember his name today. I don't remember most of those men's names. But I will call him Paul.

Before Paul's arrival I busied myself around the apartment, picking up and dusting, two of life's most relentless chores, especially for nervous gay men. But I didn't have much furniture to dust.

As is my custom on Saturday mornings, I had a telephone conversation with my mother, who lives in St. Louis. While we talked she asked me if I was nervous. *Was anything wrong?* Yes, I told her, I was a little tense, but nothing was wrong. I explained that I had joined a group of lawyers who were doing free work for guys with AIDS. I swallowed hard as I said this. We had never explicitly spoken about my being gay, but then, I figured, we had never talked about my being straight either. We just had never talked about sex; we talked around it. I told her Paul was coming to my home.

"Don't do this," she said.

"Why not?" I asked.

She didn't want to be so crass as to say what was really on her mind, so she said, "You don't know who this person is. He is a stranger; he might rob you or something."

Both of my parents had a unique talent for finding danger lurking in the most innocent of situations. While I was a child every single activity was accompanied with a caveat. Beware! Every time I left my family's house, the words "be careful" echoed after me. Even the most innocent of pastimes were fraught with a thousand dangerous possibilities. "Have fun at Disneyland but don't let anyone pick your pocket." "Don't talk to anyone." "Don't ride anything dangerous." *Don't, don't, don't...* The paradox of my parents—have fun but watch out. Later they wondered why I grew up to be so nervous.

"I don't think I have anything he could possibly want," I said.

"You might get AIDS." It was after all early in the epidemic. Most people felt the way she did. Many still do.

"Mom," I said chuckling, "I'm giving him a will, not a blow job." To this day I don't know what made me say that. Sometimes I think I'm funny in a crude way. My mother obviously didn't agree. I didn't think before I said it. My mother didn't think before she hung up on me. I was a little embarrassed. A few hours later we talked again and laughed off the incident. She's a great mom in that and many other ways.

I finished cleaning up the apartment, rehearsing everything I would need to say to Paul to do his will. I was terrified of meeting someone with AIDS but also of committing some form of malpractice. He arrived, and I tried vainly to appear at ease. In his late 30s, he was mild-mannered and dressed as if he stepped out of an L.L. Bean or J. Crew catalog. He had a pleasant face and was balding on top with a fringe of dark hair around the sides. One thing seemed clear: He did not look like a leather queen who had been promiscuous. I think this made me more nervous than I already was.

We sat together in my sparse living room to begin the process of writing his will. In the course of a will interview, a lawyer has to ask a great number of intimate and sometimes difficult questions. To try and make him comfortable at the outset, I asked if there was anything I could get for him. The snow that had been present the night of my first gay bar association meeting had given way to a sleety cold rain, the type that makes February such a difficult month for New Yorkers. I always used to say that February was the shortest month of the year out of consideration for New Yorkers. He didn't want coffee or tea, but he did ask for a glass of water, which I got for him.

During the will interview I was not terribly creative and in fact was downright clumsy. My carefully rehearsed words, which I had thought would sound sensitive and professional, now sounded strained and contrived. I wasn't acting by rote; I had never done this before, and no one in law school had ever really taught me about this part. They don't teach anything quite so practical; it is all theory. Though I felt I sounded mechanical, in the end, mostly because of his kind indulgence, it was going rather smoothly.

Then I got to the hardest part. He sat comfortably and calmly on my couch while we talked about how and to whom he wanted to distribute his property, and he told me about his family and his friends. I explained each point of the will to him, and he listened attentively. He sensed we were nearing the end of our interview.

"There's one other thing," I said.

"What's that?"

"How do you want to dispose of your bodily remains?" I hadn't been able to think of another way to say it. He appeared somewhat pained, as if I'd just walked over and slapped him across the face without warning. I felt as if I could see the red imprint of my hand on his cheek. I had tried to phrase it in a way that didn't sound so blunt, but any way I came up with still boiled down to "How do you want to dispose of your body?" Twice within a short span of time, I'd offended two people.

The moment passed. His composure had only been slightly askew. He replied that he wanted to be cremated. As it would turn out, they would almost all want to be cremated. I never knew if that was an expression about having AIDS or if it was that most of us who lived in Manhattan were keenly aware of space shortages. Some would speak of elaborate funeral arrangements, planning down to the most remote detail what exactly would happen and in what order. Those, I figured, were the real control queens. Opera fanatics were the worst because they wanted to orchestrate the whole thing, planning every detail of the service right down to what everyone would wear.

I explained to Paul what the process would be in finishing the will, we shook hands, and he left. I picked up the papers and set up the file. I tidied up, taking our glasses into the kitchen. Looking at the glass he had used, I separated it from my own. I put it in the sink by itself, put my hands on the counter, and thought about Paul dying. I experienced an involuntary shudder—someone walking over my grave. I put the tea kettle on, and when the water boiled I filled his glass with it over and over again. I felt shame for doing it, but that didn't stop me. The world after all was flat.

Eventually I finished his will, and we signed it at his apartment in Greenwich Village. He didn't sue me for malpractice. He never had the chance. I knew when he died because GMHC produced daily sheets with deceased clients' names. We called them RIP sheets. He was the first client of mine who died, and I assumed that his will went to probate without any question. But seeing his name on that RIP sheet, it became all too clear that there are just so many aspects to writing a will for someone that they just can't teach you in law school. Even though I had expected it, I took the loss of this nice guy to heart, as if his dying had let me down just a bit. I had hoped he would somehow make it. The full reality of the epidemic wasn't clear yet. That was when it was believed that not everyone with HIV would develop AIDS, and maybe not everyone with AIDS would die.

As a volunteer, I went on to do other wills. I learned a lot. For instance, not long after Paul, I asked another client how he wanted to dispose of his bodily remains. Again I inwardly writhed as I said it. It was a tough question, and it hurt to be asked it, as I'd seen on Paul's face, but it was a necessary part of the will interview. This guy was thin, drained, and pale with lesions on his body. His skin was gray and yellow. He already had a haunted expression on his face when I asked my dreaded question. His vacant and emaciated face—especially near the temples—was the classic countenance that I would later come to know as The Look. It meant that the person you were looking at wouldn't last much longer. The Look cannot be really described. It is no particular set of characteristics or combination of features. But it is not something—once you become acquainted with it—that you would confuse with anything else.

In response to my question, however, The Look melted away for a moment of fierce rage. He was furious with me. He didn't want to "dispose" of his body, he told me. It was his *body* we were talking about, not a sack of garbage. As he yelled at me, flecks of saliva erupted from his mouth in my direction. His eyes had grown wide and his fists, clenched on his lap, shook. His once vacant eyes now focused with anger on my insensitivity, and felt naked in my stupidity.

I sat there stunned and embarrassed. When he finished yelling, his anger began to melt away and he returned to the vapid, gaunt expression of before. The Look was back. That incident provides some insight into why this community is so angry. Sometimes anger is the only thing that is going to keep death away. Somehow I found my voice. I hated being yelled at like that. Somewhere a part of me wanted to say, "Look, pal, 99% of America wouldn't be caught dead even sitting in the same room with you. I'm just trying to help." I knew, however, that it wouldn't be a very helpful thing to say. He was the one dying after all, not me. He could be as angry as he wanted to be about my clumsiness. I apologized quietly. "I'm sorry." They were words that didn't seem adequate. I didn't know what to do, so I just sat there. So did he. It took him a long time to be able to talk to me again.

I learned a great and simple lesson. A will was so much about mortality and indicated so strongly the obvious—that each day you have less and less control over what is happening to your body. Terminal illness makes you as powerless as someone watching a tide go out and wanting it to come back in. I knew to make it an experience that was all right for both of us, I had to do something different—something that would make a difference in the way people perceived the whole thing.

Instead of talking about property and disposing of one's body, I began to talk about a will in terms of taking power and authority and control over rights that these men otherwise would not have as a gay person. This was especially good for gay couples. I explained how a will wasn't just about giving away property but rather to get "virtually married." When a same-sex couple leave their estates to each other and make each other executors and sign mutual powers of attorney, a couple could in effect become married by doing wills. By doing so they would get many of the same rights married couples are given automatically when they march down an aisle and say the two magic words "I do." That made the will more about taking back rights than about dying and leaving property.

And whenever I asked a client about the disposition of his or her bodily remains as part of the will, I always took the time to talk about myself first. No one ever seemed uncomfortable again, when I put it in those terms. I explained that the main reason I had done a will is that I wanted to express my wishes about being cremated, because I absolutely did not want to be buried. Did you have any wishes like that? That approach worked better, but personalizing the issue created other questions.

"Are you sick too?" they might ask.

"No," I would say, embarrassed. "I'm not." It would not be the last time I was embarrassed to admit that I wasn't sick.

"You don't know what it's like then," they might say.

"Even if I were sick," I learned to say, "I wouldn't know exactly what it is like for you."

These conversations served to intensify my own personal fears—the ones that came to me like a stalker's phone call late at night. "Are you sick too?" It was a tough question, a relative question. Did I have the virus? There was still no test, and even if there were, I would be too afraid to take it. I would lie in bed at night and wonder and worry that if I were sick, it would be so hard for my family. I did not know what I could do to make it easier for them. I wondered if they were worried that I might be sick. I wondered if they talked about it with each other. I wondered if they wanted to talk about it with me but were afraid or embarrassed.

The other wills were also for people who died quickly, but unlike Paul, they did not do the will between bouts of opportunistic infections. Rather, it was at the last minute, when they were on their deathbeds. I had to work my way up to doing deathbed wills. It had to be approached cautiously. Doing a regular will for someone with AIDS—that was a bunny hill. Doing a deathbed will was like skiing down a steep mountain and seeing that just ahead a few yards, there was no more snow. I was never very comfortable with death. At first I always turned the opportunity to do deathbed wills down flat, telling Steve to find someone else. He understood completely. I was so very terrified of being next to a hospital bed while someone was dying. It wasn't their mortality I was afraid of; it was mine.

My experience with death had been so limited, as it normally is for young people. My grandfather died of a heart attack when I was 7 years old and it was very sudden. My family knew he was dead for a whole day before they told me. But my first real experience had been the year before that when I was 6 years old and my grandfather's aunt died in her sleep. I had met her only once a few months before her death, but she had been very kind to me. We were in her home. It was the home of an elderly woman—with dark furniture, glass-paned doors, and doilies laid over everything from couches to end tables. She was the quintessential old lady, complete with gray hair pulled back into a bun and pleasant blue eyes. She was as unaccustomed to entertaining people my age as I was of being entertained by someone as old as she, so while she had no milk and cookies to offer me, she gave me crackers and water. It was a hot day and I didn't want crackers and water, but I knew she wanted to please me and I was loathe to hurt her feelings. I suffered through eating those dry crackers and drinking that warm tap water, as eager to please her as she had been to please me. Not long after that day, she died. It was the first I knew of death, and I was extremely upset when my parents told me that we were going to her funeral. I thought how unfair it was for this kind and gentle lady to die. Where did she go, I asked? What happened to her? Why did this happen? I may have been only 6 years old, but over all this time I find my questions then are the same ones I have today, and they remain unanswered. And the same sense of unfairness pervades my questions. I cried so hard when we went to the funeral that my parents had to remove me.

Now the rooms where these boys died were invariably hot. Strange, repugnant odors filled my nostrils. I witnessed the indignities of an adult forced to wear diapers, attached to a catheter with hollowed-out cheeks and yellowed skin. It seemed sometimes as if human frailty and decline had a common scent. Seeing someone dying of AIDS was at first too much for me to handle. I was too embarrassed for them and for me. I was too afraid for them and for me. It was too unfair. Where were they going? And I didn't think I was up to the pretense of pretending I was enjoying my dry crackers and warm tap water any more.

## DEATH BE NOT PROUD

My father died in 1980 of lung cancer. I made two trips to St. Louis to see him. The first time, when he was diagnosed, he looked like he had a bad cold. Four months later, when I went to say good-bye, he weighed only about 90 pounds, and he had tumors all over his body. He was a bit demented from the brain tumors. He would not even look at me when I said good-bye.

But the experience had taught me something very valuable. Up to the time I saw my father dying of cancer, I was always imagining that I had cancer. A pain in one side of my body meant liver cancer, a pain in another side meant pancreatic cancer. When I was 13 I read *Death Be Not Proud,* by the parents of a young man who died of brain cancer, and I had been convinced for months that every headache was a brain tumor. I obsessed about it. All that ended when I saw my father. Seeing someone really die of cancer diminished my fear of it considerably. Rarely would I ever again imagine that I had cancer because I had become so well-acquainted with it I now knew what it was really like. For a while I began to live normally, not paranoically thinking that every ache in my side, every shortness of breath was cancer. That was a brief luxury I enjoyed just before the AIDS epidemic.

The new demon that rushed forth to take its place was, of course, AIDS. I was always sure that at any moment on any morning I might wake up short of breath or I might find a purple Karposi's sarcoma lesion on my leg. Every mark on my body was examined thoroughly. I was not alone in this type of paranoia. AIDS paranoia, in fact, became a standard lifestyle for many gay men. I heard a story in New York about one man who had several moles on his body. His lover photographed his entire body so that they could tell if there was anything unusual occurring. I cannot claim any exceptional level of neurosis on this point. It didn't make a difference that I hadn't been promiscuous; non-promiscuous people were dying. It only mattered that I was gay. And each day I woke up wondering if this would be the day that the shortness of breath would come, that the lesion would appear. It became not a matter of *if* but *when*. There were always comments, whispered stories at social gatherings, ear bent to mouth about this person or that guy.

"He had slept with only five people in his whole life."

"He had never had anal intercourse."

"They were in a monogamous relationship, and they were both diagnosed."

Hearing these secret murmurings at a meeting or a party or a chance encounter with a friend on the subway was like hearing an air-raid siren in the distance. It didn't just mean trouble. It meant that you should be afraid. Be afraid before anything else. Take cover. Run. Hide. Put your head down and run.

# CHAPTER 4 : 1984

---

*6,130 new cases of AIDS were diagnosed*
*3,436 more people died*
*A cumulative total of 10,683 cases were diagnosed*
*5,502 people were dead of AIDS in America*

---

## LEARNING LESSONS

On some instinctual level maybe I knew that doing a deathbed will was probably going to be a good thing for me. Still, the merest memory of a hospital and the experience of seeing my father suffer the effects of a catastrophic illness evoked so much fear of death and, worse, pain. But one day Mother Teresa, Esq., called me for a deathbed-will situation in my neighborhood. He hadn't been able to get anyone else. I don't know if this was Providence or Accident. Whatever it was, I went.

Today I don't remember a thing about that first one. I don't remember who it was for, which hospital it was at, or even what he looked like. It's like trying to remember the first time I had to swim. I don't remember doing that either, but I know it must have happened because I can swim now.

Whenever and wherever and for whomever it was, I did it. And then I began to do them more often. Steve called on me more and more frequently. I actually became good at it, so good that Steve began calling me whenever he had a deathbed will situation that he couldn't handle himself.

I never stopped being afraid, though. And after the many dozens that I did, I still don't think I could walk into the room of a person covered with KS lesions who was sucking in the breath of a respirator and not feel the sweat running down my spine. It happened every time. Today whenever I walk into a hospital to visit with a sick friend, I feel claustrophobic and I want to run. I don't know what I would do if I had to be a patient in a hospital myself.

Being afraid was in a way the good part. It kept me going back to one after another. As much as it terrified me I found I was also struck by a sense of awe when I found that I could look at the situation, gauge my fear, and then go ahead and do it anyway. To this day, staring down that fear is the most empowering thing I have ever done in my life. I don't mean anything heroic about this. It wasn't heroism. Something compelling cannot be termed heroic. I walked into those sweaty godforsaken deathbed rooms because I was doing it for me. It was my best defense against my enemy AIDS. It was my discovery that I was more powerful than my worst fears. Perhaps it was nothing more than discovering that I had been afraid of cancer before, but now there was AIDS. I had been afraid of a dog, but now I saw the lion. The dog no longer had any power over me.

In 1984 hundreds of thousands of Americans already were infected with HIV, as yet undiscovered. However, at this time there were only a few thousand people living with AIDS in the United States. Most of them were in Los Angeles, San Francisco, and New York. And there was no HIV antibody test. The volunteer lawyers of the pro bono panel therefore often met their clients on a trip to the hospital—a trip that might be a first for the volunteer and the last for the client.

There was one deathbed will I did that remains special and distinct for me. Many of those trips have now by the grace of some safety mechanism faded into one another, melting together, filed away in my brain under the heading Bad Time—Don't Look Too Deeply. But there are some individuals I do remember. There was one in particular in Lenox Hill Hospital with an incredibly obnoxious lover who became so intrusive and odious that I had to insist he leave the room during our consultations.

The man's will was drafted, but he put off signing the thing until he was in the hospital and on his deathbed. We had to coordinate witnesses, finding friends who knew him best and could attest to the fact that he was not demented at the time of the will signing. I met them for the first time when I got to the hospital. They were nervous and uncomfortable. I tried to put them at ease by being matter of fact about what we had to do. This occurred in the "old days" of the epidemic, when hospitals made you suit up with a mask, a gown, and gloves—and for the most cautious, a little cap—before going into a PWA's room.

*PWA* stands for *person with AIDS*. That is the preferred terminology, even though the media were hell-bent on calling them AIDS victims for purposes of convenience, even though that represented something repugnant to PWAs. I could never understand why the media would never bend on this. Black people didn't want to be called Negroes anymore, and the media respected that. But they call PWAs "AIDS victims." With respect to something as foreign to them as AIDS in general, the media could not get its act together to objectively report what was going on in the epidemic. Unfortunately, while so many things in AIDS have changed rapidly, this has not. Members of the media, including lesbian and gay journalists working for large metropolitan dailies, still either don't get it or have editors who don't.

I walked into Lenox Hill and found the appointed room. I would walk down those hallways, secretly stealing glances into rooms. Even the feet sticking outside their covers looked sick. Coughs and moans echoed in the hallway. I would take particular note of how many of the rooms had warning signs posted outside them. In the earliest days they said AIDS, but later they just warned that bodily fluid precautions had to be used when entering the room—i.e., suiting up. Outside the hospital room the witnesses and I suited up in our paper-and-plastic protective fashions. It used to be that when policemen would arrest AIDS activists, they too would wear these little outfits. A lot of the boys would taunt them with phrases like "Your gloves don't match your gown!" or with shouts of "No gloves without pearls before 5!" Soon the police began to switch to just gloves.

This day in Lenox Hill I joked with the witnesses that we all looked like we were ready to do a Playtex commercial. They laughed and felt more at ease. I smiled back, but I did not feel any more at ease.

The little "ceremony" of a will signing is prescribed by the statute that covers this subject. It is designed to serve as proof that a person signing a will has mental capacity and is aware of what he or she is doing and is doing it by free will. The person signing the will is asked a series of questions by the presiding attorney.

"Is this your will?"

"Have you read it?"

"Do you understand and agree with its contents?"

"Does it reflect your wishes?"

"Would you please ask these people to witness your will?"

The testator then puts his or her initials on each page of the will and signs it, asking the witnesses in turn to sign it. Then it is done.

When we got up next to the hospital bed, my heart sank. He was awake but had no strength, and he was having trouble staying awake. He was moving and his eyes would open, but he didn't really seem alive to me. He was older than I was by about 20 years, which made me glad. I needed to put a lot of distance between him and me.

*Oh, God,* I thought, *if I am ever like this, please just have someone put a pillow over my face and bring me to a merciful end.*

Clearly he would not be able to read the will, so I would have to read it to him. The sound of my voice passively enunciating his wishes in the passionless prose of the will was the only sound in the room except for the whirring of hospital machinery pumping medicine, pumping oxygen, measuring heartbeats.

Suddenly there was a commotion at the door. His family had shown up and were trying to get into the room. They were seemingly hostile to the will and everyone else. I got up and asked them to leave. I no sooner began to recite the will once more when the lover showed up.

"Has he signed yet?"

"No," I said with undisguised contempt, "he hasn't. And it is in your own best interests not to be here." He left, and I returned to the will.

Then a nurse arrived with an EKG unit announcing that she had to do this procedure then and there. I could not imagine the need for doing an EKG on a dying man but politely explained to her that we were in the middle of signing his will and asked if she might come back later.

In a clear and decisive manner, she flatly said no. She said it would have to be now or not at all. I peered at her over my mask, feeling like Jack Nicholson in *Five Easy Pieces*. "Well then, honey, guess what," I said. "It's going to be not at all." I stuck my head out the door and called to the nurses station, and they came and got the EKG nurse to change her mind. With hostile nurse, hostile family, and hostile lover now safely outside, I shut and barred the door and went on with the process necessary under New York law to administer a proper will signing. Sweat poured out of me as if a faucet inside had been turned to full throttle, soaking my clothes underneath the cap and gown and goggles and gloves. I felt like a priest determined to marry a couple with the entire world holding objection.

I looked back to the client who was still in the same position in his bed. His mouth gaped open like a newborn bird waiting for feeding. I wasn't sure that he had followed everything that had happened. He obviously wanted to sleep. It occurred to me what a circus this must all be to him. Lying there dying with at least a dozen dysfunctional people around him all with their own agendas, few of which really had to do with him. If I were he, I would have resented this intrusion into my death.

The witnesses were beginning to melt fast with fatigue and emotion. My own veneer of professional demeanor began to let me down. I wanted to make sure that my client was awake. I looked at him and tugged on his thin arm and took his face in my hand. He was a tall and gangly man, looking nothing at all like me physically. He was older and gray and, of course, frail—so frail that he could barely move.

"Do you understand everything that's happened here?"

He nodded.

"Can you answer me?"

He nodded.

"Then answer me!"

The witnesses looked at me as if I had turned from Dr. Jekyll to Mr. Hyde. But I had an obligation to make sure that he was cogent before letting him sign the will.

So that I didn't look so ghoulish, I added a gentle and tentative "OK?"

"Uh-huh."

"Good."

As I let go of his face I could very clearly see myself sitting there in that bed, dying. This was my looking glass, my crystal ball. I knew that one day I would be there too, dying. Inside I could feel myself even now dying. I didn't know if I was infected. But I thought surely I would be dying here too.

"Do you remember me reading your will?" He nodded.

"Do you?" I asked again sharply.

"Yes."

"Did it reflect your wishes? You are sure it is what you want?" I had worked so long to get this man to sign his will before going into the hospital, and he had never wavered on the contents of the will at all.

He nodded again. Then he said "Uh-huh." And then finally it came time to sign the instrument. I put the pen in his hand and it slid out. I put it in again and it slid out again. Witnesses began to cry. I hated it when they couldn't sign. But the clever and resourceful New York legislature foresaw this and the statute accounts for this possibility.

It meant, however, that I would have to hoist my body up next to him, half lying in his bed with him. I put my arm around him and my masked face next to his, and through my gloved hand I held his hand, which in turn held the pen. Together very slowly we wrote his name.

The witnesses, a man and two women, began to cry harder. I did not. They then signed their names as witnesses, and it was over. I made sure the client was comfortable. I thanked him and told him he had done a good job. He closed his eyes. He was headed for the finish line now.

We went outside and said good-bye to one another. The hallway was now deserted. Timing really is everything. I congratulated them on a job well-done. I went to the nurses' station still suited up and asked where the nearest place was where I could get rid of my suit. I went to a lavatory and looked in the mirror. I saw myself, but in my mind I also saw him in his bed. I felt like I had aged 15 years in 15 minutes. I removed my cap and gown and then my gloves. I looked at them and thought about what a ridiculous waste of money this was. They make us wear this while he is in the hospital, and if he were discharged, he'd take a cab home or ride the subway, and no on would be wearing a cap or gown. It was so stupid. I decided I wasn't going to wear them anymore. I went to the sink and began to splash cold water on my face to sober myself up again.

The gloves contain a resin of some kind, a sort of fine powdery substance that ensures against slippage for people doing medical procedures as they perspire inside the gloves. The resin, or whatever it is, had a distinct odor that clung stubbornly to one's hands. When I had washed my hands with soap, I held my fingers to my nose to find that the smell hadn't dissipated. I washed them again and held them to my nose a second time. Still, I could smell the rank odor of that resin. But it didn't smell like resin. To me it smelled exactly like a decaying body. I tried again—this time in earnest—and began to scrub and scrub and scrub furiously, and still when I finished I lifted my hands to my nose and could still smell it. I could smell the odor from a funeral home on my hands. As I washed again, I began to cry.

I was still wet in my clothes from the perspiration that came along with the confrontation with the nurse, the closeness of his dying body on mine, of being suited up. And I could not control the crying. I had wits enough to know that I ought to leave the hospital, so I quickly walked out of the bathroom and down a set of stairs and tried to leave. But when I got to the doors to the street, I found I was terrified of walking outside. I got right up to the doors but could not walk out. I backed away from the doors, walking instead around the corridor, crying, wringing my hands like Lady MacBeth. Then I tried a second time to go out and again found myself held back by the sheer terror of going outside. My vale of tears was beginning to attract attention in the lobby, so I ducked into a telephone booth next to the entrance.

There, between violent sobs, I managed to do one of the most sensible things I have ever done. For once in my life I had a quarter when I needed it, and I telephoned Gay Men's Health Crisis, asking for one of the therapists on staff there. He came on the line, quickly assessing my terror and asked me if I would come down to see him. I looked at the doors to the hospital and began to choke on a sob again and said no. I explained to him that I was suddenly afraid to leave the hospital, to go out onto the street, to get out of the phone booth. I was afraid that the inevitable was going to happen to me. I knew that I was going to die of AIDS as surely as that man upstairs. Chuck, the therapist, asked me why I couldn't go outside, but I didn't know why. I could only repeat that I was afraid to go out.

"Can't you get on the subway?" he asked.

"No, absolutely not. Not the subway." The thought of being in a crush of people made my stomach turn. The stark contrast between the world out there and the world in this hospital was more than a door could separate. The people out there had no idea what was going on in here.

After that I really don't remember what he said to me, but he was very gentle and very good. Something in whatever he said made me feel that this little breakdown I was having was perfectly logical under the circumstances; he convinced me that it was totally within my power to go out the door and to get into a cab and ride down from the east side to 18th Street, where GMHC was located. He said he would be there on the street ready to talk to me. I went outside, and my luck that began with finding a quarter for the telephone held out, and with the grace of God I found a cab. I still cried all the way. Now, the greatest thing in the world in this kind of situation is a New York cab driver. They've seen everything, and you can't impress or scare them. When I arrived, Chuck was there, true to his word. We talked for an hour. I told him that I was afraid of becoming the man in that bed. I was afraid there would be no one left to care for me. And then, feeling better, the next day I did two deathbed wills. It was the only time I ever suffered that kind of paralyzing breakdown, although I did cry sometimes in hospitals after that.

I had been raised to believe that only people who were ill used therapists and that it was a sign of emotional and mental weakness. In one afternoon, a lifetime of such conditioning was completely dismantled and replaced by a deep-seated respect and reverence for good therapy. Now to my mind, going into therapy, either short- or long-term, is a symbol of strength, of a commitment to finding things in one's makeup that are rough-edged and making them smooth. It is work, it is commitment, and it is an act of strength, not weakness, and it had taken me a long time to understand that. But it was over in an hour.

## WORST NIGHTMARE

As galvanizing as this experience was, it was still not the most memorable for me. It was one of the first situations I have ever encountered with a person confined to a bed who was devastated by the ravages of an illness that the press still didn't cover. An illness for which we didn't know the cause, that seemed to be aiming its sights at people all around me. And I was braced to receive my first bullet. Every morning I busied myself by performing a body check in the shower, making careful mental notes of my breathing patterns while jogging around the reservoir in Central Park.

Today, so many years later, a walk around Manhattan will still bring to mind for me many of the deathbed wills I used to do. I can point out apartment buildings where I had to go, as if conducting some macabre kind of architectural walking tour. No matter what time of year it was, it was always so damned hot in the rooms where people were on their deathbeds, or maybe it just made me sweat a lot.

These experiences taught me two of the most important lessons of my life. The first lesson: Looking into the mouth of hell teaches you something important. After a while of looking at it, it just can't scare you anymore. It just begins to lose its power. I don't believe in hell anymore. Hell isn't a place; it's a state of mind. Hell is something you go through but not a place you visit. My arrival at this conclusion is one of the worthwhile lessons of all my years of AIDS work. Without having gone through the experiences I have, I don't know that I would have arrived at the same conclusion. I think I would have lived my life like I was before, afraid of so many unknown shadows lurking in the corners of my imagination. Afraid of hell. But there is no such place. Hell is fear, nothing more or less.

In 1984 the fear that clung the hardest to me was my fear of Kaposi's sarcoma. The second lesson: People who have nothing left to lose are in the best position to overcome their worst fears. KS is a difficult opportunistic infection to accept for a number of reasons. It can be disfiguring. A rare skin cancer usually found among elderly Mediterranean men, it began appearing more and more in the cases I saw. It was insidious, attacking noses and ears, making once-beautiful faces discolored, swollen, and hideous. It attacked limbs, forming tumors that cut off circulation. It could go inside and attack organs and eyes, causing them to cease functioning. It was the meanest opportunistic infection I then thought could exist. As it turns out, I was wrong about that. There are other infections that no one had heard about in 1984 but that began to occur with frequency in the 1990s; diseases such as progressive multifocal leukoencephalopathy, which is like a combination of Lou Gehrig's disease and Alzheimer's in its effect but which is swifter than either. I have seen PML reduce a beautiful athlete to a vegetative, bedridden state in as little as four months. But in 1984 PWAs rarely survived long enough to get any opportunistic infection besides Kaposi's sarcoma and *Pneumocystis carinii* pneumonia.

I was called to the home of a man named Richard for a deathbed signing. The door was opened by a tall, handsome, well-built man with mild manners that had been taught him by a careful mother somewhere in the Midwest. He was prematurely graying a bit. He escorted me into the living room beyond him, where, of course, it was stifling hot. No one else seemed to notice. In the center of the room, facing away from the door, was a hospital bed with a large man in it. He was barely wearing any pajamas, although his torso was covered. There were other men—his care partners—in the room.

I walked around the room, meeting everyone, and turned to face the man who was propped up in the bed. It appeared as if he had no skin. Richard's eyes met mine from a pool of swollen red scabs that distorted his features. It was impossible to tell what he had once looked like. The scabs and lesions traveled down his powerfully girded arms; his bare legs, both propped up on pillows, were unnaturally swollen masses of decaying flesh. There was a nauseating smell of decay. Richard had little or none of his nose left. He was literally rotting away.

I had never imagined that KS could take so much of a person without first killing him. But apparently Richard's internal organs were untouched. He still had a hearty appetite and was not weak. The man who had opened the door for me, Allen Wallace, told me that Richard ate like a horse and had no other AIDS problems—just the KS. Later under different circumstances Allen and I would meet again. He would become one of my dearest friends.

Richard's eyes never left mine. He scrutinized me carefully for my reaction to his appearance. I wish I could say that I handled this so well that we were all laughing by the end of it. But I was nervous. My eyes had to have widened a bit. I know I trembled slightly. But as much as I wanted to stare at anything else in the room, I tried not to let my eyes leave Richard's. Allen introduced me to Richard. I put my hand out to grasp his, and we shook. It took a lot of effort on my part not to wipe my hand on my pants, not to shiver, and not to look away. Nevertheless, I hated myself for what weakness was showing through. I felt like Richard hated me for it too. His eyes returned a challenging gaze as if he were daring me—to see how long I could look at him without an overt signal of my revulsion.

We didn't really speak; he merely acknowledged my recitation of the instruments I had brought for him to sign. I got through it as quickly as possible and said good-bye to everyone. I purposefully shook Richard's hand good-bye, meeting his gaze as best I could. I wanted to get out of that room quickly. I wanted to deny that such things actually were happening. I left, and though I don't remember, I am sure that I got drunk. A few days later I heard that Richard's legs were amputated. I never saw him again—at least not in person. The memory of Richard will stay with me always. I never saw before or since a case of KS that looked like that. I hope I never see anything like it again. He lived for a good many months after that day.

I remember uttering the words "Thank God" when I saw Richard's name on my RIP sheet. However, Richard's face would visit me many times after that. Late at night lying alone in my bed, his eyes would stare again into my own with his challenging expression while I lay wondering if there was a virus in my body eating away my immune system, waiting to steal my youth and looks and happiness away from me as it had done to Richard. Each time it happened, I tried to push him further and further away. But Richard will never, ever leave me.

## A CLOSE CALL

One day not long after that while getting ready for work in the morning, I felt something unusual in my mouth. I ran my tongue over it and discovered a lump. I met my own eyes in the bathroom mirror and asked myself whether I was ready to face whatever this might be. I aimed my face upward into the light and pulled my mouth open with my finger but was unable to see clearly. I found a flashlight and shone it into my reflection. There it was, just as I knew it would be: a purple lesion about the size of a dime. There was no question in my mind what it was. A feeling of panic washed over me almost simultaneously with a feeling of relief—relief that it had begun, that I no longer had to wait to discover it. Then too I felt dread of the awful, disfiguring, and painful death I would have.

On my way to the doctor I wondered how I would tell my family. I knew that they would suffer a great deal over this. After a nervous and paralyzing wait, I got in to see my doctor, and he examined the lesion.

"Have you been nervous lately?" he asked.

"Wouldn't you be?"

"Before, I mean. Have you been under any stress lately?"

It seemed pointless to rattle off the feelings of stress I had associated with doing these wills, of watching what was happening to people.

"Yeah," I said, "I've been under stress."

"Well," he said calmly, "it shows. You've chewed a hole in the wall of your mouth and bruised it terribly. But you don't have KS."

I let out a breath of relief and felt my consciousness return to normal, only to wait for the next time.

There was a next time and a time after that. Like many friends, I made several trips to the doctor based on false alarms. They were not all alike, because after one of the trips the doctor and I started dating. Nothing felt safer than dating a doctor. It would at least cut down on the trips across town I'd have to make when I could just ask from across the bed, "Honey, is this a KS lesion?"

1 9 8 4

## PEOPLE IN THE PARK

In the early spring of 1984 I found that I needed a little break from the routine. I was now a regular volunteer for Steve Gittleson, who was on staff at GMHC as director of legal services. It had been a cold and snowy winter, and I had had my first really miserable experiences and gotten past them. One morning while I was at work at the investment firm, I had a sudden urge. I telephoned Rodger McFarlane, who was no longer just an ex-neighbor but a good friend and even mentor.

"I need to get away," I said. "I was thinking it would be fun to go to Puerto Rico for the weekend. Wanna go?" I worked in the Seagram building at 53rd Street and Park Avenue. I gazed longingly from my office window out toward the distant airports.

"Baby, are you crazy?" he asked. "I have a responsible position here. This place is a virtual powder keg from minute to minute. One of my staff members just got diagnosed, and the whole goddamned staff is hysterical. I can't just up and go to Puerto Rico for the weekend just because you're having a bad day," he said.

I felt bad. Everything he described sounded pretty horrible, and there I was sitting in my ivory (Seagram) tower in my corner office, wanting a weekend at the beach. I'd never been to Puerto Rico.

"It was just a fleeting thought," I said. "It seemed like a good idea when I thought of it."

We hung up, and I looked out at the airports for a good, long while, wondering where all those planes were going and pretending that I was on one. Twenty minutes later my phone rang. It was Rodger. He had made reservations, and we would leave Friday morning.

We made a rule about this trip. No one could say the "A word," and we managed the weekend without violating this pact for the most part—except for when Rodger suggested that I join the board of directors of a small AIDS organization in the city that was trying to provide housing for people with AIDS. The AIDS Resource Center had a small board of directors and a few volunteers. Included on the board was a great woman, the Rev. Lee Hancock of Greenwich Village's Judson Church.

Lee is a woman of vision who lets her spirit guide her and who turns her ideals into her reality. That is, I have come to find, a rare gift. Lee is one of the most genuine people I have ever met. It is difficult not to sound corny when describing her, but it is easy to see that the grace of God lives in Lee. It was not possible for me to meet her without falling in love with her.

When we got back from Puerto Rico and Rodger introduced me, that is what happened—I fell in love with her. In the course of an hour I felt I'd known her all my life. She invited me to a few ARC board meetings, held in a dreary basement room in a brownstone in Chelsea that smelled occasionally of sewage. ARC had been in existence for over a year by then and had raised over $50,000. Its mandate was to house people who had become homeless because of AIDS—but as yet it had housed no one. I joined the board and the group of well-intentioned extremely disparate people, and together we sat looking at the problem of homelessness and wondering how to solve it.

Housing in New York is one of the toughest challenges for anyone, from the east-side millionaire to the unemployed homeless person. Over the years I've heard many stories about people looking for apartments: paying huge sums of money as finder's fees and key money to agents and building supers, waking up at 5 A.M. on Wednesday to buy a *Village Voice* for the classifieds, and even scouring obituaries for the names of people who had died and then looking up their apartment to see when it was becoming available. There is no New York story about apartment hunting that is too wild to be true.

For a newcomer to the city, finding a place to live is the most intimidating and discouraging thing about the city. For a person who had lost his job and his friends because he had this new disease, the challenge could be insurmountable. For the rich, it is a matter of finding the right apartment. For the middle class, it is simply a matter of getting the best space for the most reasonable amount of money, which is usually not much for a lot. For the poor, finding housing in New York means finding something in a neighborhood that is not safe in the bright of day, is a walk-up of four or five stories, or living in a single-resident occupancy. An SROs can be scary just to walk by. They are monuments to urban despair. Near my first apartment in New York on 81st and Broadway, there were two SROs, or welfare hotels, that smelled so badly of urine that I would trot as I passed them on my way to the park, especially on a hot day. The dank smell of urine came across like a tangible form of hopelessness. Today both of those welfare hotels are expensive condominiums.

Back in those days we looked at homelessness through a lens of AIDS because the disease caused a financial spiral downward, leaving people unable to afford a place to live. Later in the epidemic we would need to flip that lens and look at how AIDS is effecting chronic homelessness. Unfortunately, hardly anyone has done that.

The AIDS Resource Center was in serious trouble. Without any paid staff, the board of directors had to do most of the work, and the work involved trying to keep our heads above water. Consequently, there were board meetings that would last as long as five excruciating hours. Some of the board members were unemployed and so had a great deal of time on their hands. Some, like Lee, were ministers or ministry students, since ARC was also founded with a strong spiritual base. The original $50,000 the organization held had soon gone toward office rent, legal expenses, and putting on small fund-raisers that cost more than they took in. It was gone, and before long the board was at the point of having to chip in contributions so that we could come up with the office rent. The thought that someone would ever be housed by this organization seemed in doubt when we could barely house ourselves.

*11,581 new cases of AIDS were diagnosed*
*6,831 more people died*
*A cumulative total of 22,274 cases were diagnosed in America*
*12,333 people were dead of AIDS in America*

Lee and I became cochairs of the AIDS Resource Center. We began by making a commitment that no board meeting would last more than two hours and vowing that we would begin to house people. Our second big task was, with no money at all in the bank, to hire an executive director. Once that decision was made, our luck began to change. I wrote four four-page letters to various churches—including my own, the Riverside Church, where the Rev. William Sloane Coffin was minister—asking for support, which resulted in $22,000 in contributions. Reverend Coffin came through. Stamps cost 22 cents in those days, so for 88 cents we got a good return. We also began writing grant proposals. City money became available for AIDS, and we applied for it, still with nowhere to house people. There still was no federal money being spent on AIDS.

Now with about $20,000 in the bank and a new executive director, we tried our hand at fund-raising again. We secured a night at the Limelight, a popular church turned disco in Chelsea. It was a show and a dance with appearances by Harvey Fierstein, Maurice Hines, and miraculously, Whoopi Goldberg, who was one of the most generous and gracious people I've ever met. Lee's husband had connections in the entertainment industry and had been able to secure the entertainment and lighting and even arrange for the tickets. We had press coverage with local television stations covering the event—AIDS fund-raisers were big news back then—but we were never sure of how many tickets were sold nor how many people would show up. I obsessed over this. I walked into the place in the beginning, and no one was there. It was my worst fear realized, and I got so upset that I went to the bathroom and threw up. Maurice Hines kindly got me a drink. I went back into the room an hour later, and it was packed with people. We raised several thousand dollars. Still, we had housed no one.

Then one day a woman contacted the office. She had several apartments available in a building in Chelsea that she would consider renting to us for a cut rate. She said she wanted to do the right thing but was nervous about it and needed to learn more about AIDS. She had contacted the Centers for Disease Control in Atlanta for information, but I also visited her in her home. She talked to her children about it, and upon reflection she felt that this was something she could do. It is remarkable to consider the fact that this woman found it in herself to do this when a short time later Ryan White and the Ray family would both experience discrimination by their entire towns. Ryan

White and the Ray family both had to move away, the Rays having had their home set on fire because two of the Rays' sons were infected with HIV.

The board got very excited. After being in existence for over three years, it looked like we were going to be able to house someone. We began to do outreach for candidates, but it didn't take much outreach. People with AIDS who got sick, lost their job, had no insurance, and whose families who wouldn't take them back, were becoming homeless quickly and were growing in number. We drew up a lease and got it ready for signature. Late at night in my bed I would think about signing that lease for the organization and was too excited to sleep.

Working on the board of ARC had been a great deal of struggle for everyone involved, and to get one of these guys into an apartment for the end of his life was going to make it all worthwhile. There was a man who had been a composer and a saxophone player who, though he had at one time been successful, had just hocked his saxophone for money and needed a place to live. Finally everything was in place, we had a date for signing the lease, and I was going to buy champagne for the board meeting at which Lee and I would sign it. But the evening of the meeting came, and we met in our dank basement and signed the lease for the first housing project in New York City for people with AIDS in a rather cheerless fashion, without ceremony. Somehow we were tired by that first lease. It was hard for me to understand why the board felt blue, but I think we realized that this represented not the end but the beginning. It was a tough realization, and it didn't call for champagne.

With that first lease we housed 13 people, which felt like a great victory in the wake of all our financial problems. We looked to open two more and identified properties on which we would be signing two new leases. We were working particularly hard in this regard—a gay couple had been identified to us who were both sick with AIDS and were living in Central Park.

I was thunderstruck by that. I couldn't imagine being so unloved by the world—to be left in a park to die. It was unfathomable. My own family would never let such a thing happen to one of us. I thought of these two men, once the small children of someone, somewhere. Not even in their mid 20s, they faced unknown pain and suffering with a disease that brought something bizarre every day, and they were left to live in a park. It was not that the concept of homeless people was new to me; I was after all living in New York. But the homeless people I saw were chronically poor, mentally ill, or had drifted into poverty by reason of alcoholism or drug addiction. But the idea that someone who might have a job one day would be homeless the next day simply because he was ill was something I didn't think could happen in America. Such was and is my naïveté, because I still have trouble grasping it.

Helping those two men get into a home became an integral part of the drive to finish the two new leases. But a few days before the transaction was finalized, one of the men died in the park, and the other went to Boston. In their place we were able to house a man who had AIDS and his retarded, pregnant wife. "Sometimes," I wrote that night in my diary, "I feel my heart break a little more every day."

## BOWING ON THE STAGE
## OF THE METROPOLITAN OPERA
## WITHOUT SINGING A NOTE

Later in that year ARC was offered the chance to share in a fund-raiser with the AIDS Medical Foundation and the Gay Men's Health Crisis. The AMF, headed by Dr. Mathilde Krim, was the forerunner of the American Foundation for AIDS Research, before its merger with the West Coast group that was formed by Elizabeth Taylor in response to Rock Hudson's AIDS diagnosis. AMF met with early fund-raising successes through many of the contacts of Dr. Krim and her husband, Arthur Krim, head of Orion Pictures. GMHC was fast becoming a successful and sophisticated fund-raising organization, and its leaders decided to reach out to the fledgling ARC when they were holding a gala night at the Metropolitan Opera.

The evening would benefit GMHC, AMF, and ARC. The list of performers was incredible for that time. Bette Midler and Lily Tomlin, to name a few, were among the entertainment for the show, produced by Barry Brown and Fritz Holt. The evening was called "The Best of the Best."

The genesis of this show occurred while Rodger was the executive director of GMHC, and he worked hard pulling together all the parties to make the show a reality—it was a rare kind of vision in those days. More people were involved than I would know of, but Actors' Equity was key and, I suspect, provided much of the glue for the event. We worked with the organizations for months. As it would turn out, during the show the head of each of the organizations would be introduced at various points to the audience. Dr. Krim would bow for AMF, new executive director Richard Dunne would bow for GMHC, and I would get to take a bow for ARC. Knowing there was not a chance in hell I would ever again be on the stage of the Metropolitan Opera, I sought out my coworker Christopher Clark for advice. I spent more money than I originally had on my tuxedo by purchasing a cummerbund made of black sequins and beads. We didn't actually get on the stage but had a spot light on our seat while we stood and waved. That night we raised more than $1 million, breaking a record and shattering the million-dollar ceiling for the first time at an AIDS fund-raiser on the East Coast.

I think back often to those two guys in the park and the anticlimax in signing that lease to house the first people with AIDS in New York. I wonder if there is anyone else to remember them. I wonder how many more have died in the park. The excitement of the organization's finally making it and the payoff of everyone's hard work was such a contrast to our dour and somber mood at that board meeting where we signed the first lease. We did not enjoy a sense of accomplishment, and this in some ways became the typical mood for all our community efforts at building AIDS organizations. Our success is only a symbol of our failures. Our success, good as it might be, stops few from dying. But now, with several hundred thousand dollars in the bank and a network of housing units located in various apartment buildings, ARC was launched. Today it is one of the three largest AIDS organizations in New York. That was a special night, not only getting to take my bow at the Met—or watching all those celebrities turn out in 1985 for AIDS and seeing everyone's hard work pay off—it was the knowledge that we had finally made it as an organization. And the evening proved to be the benchmark for AIDS fund-raisers in the future. Rodger, Fritz, Barry, and all the willing star power had planned a hell of a show, and they took that vision and ran with it. It was exciting to watch from the audience, realizing that you were watching more than singing and dancing but a consciousness-raising, historic event that would revolutionize the way the entertainment industry approached AIDS. We were no longer a charity stepchild.

After the show there was a dinner party at the Met. I gushed more than a bit when Colleen Dewhurst came up to me and with both of my hands in hers thanked me for my work. But throughout the party I had a nagging undertow of melancholy despite our success that night. Maybe it was a postpartum depression, the letdown of something being over after anticipating it for so long. But then again maybe the worst thing about that night for me was the sense that once more what felt like an end was in fact only a beginning.

## ANOTHER CLOSE CALL

A psychologist with whom I had for some time been flirting, finally asked me out. He came to pick me up, brought flowers, and said all the right things. We had a wonderful time, and he spent the night. In the morning while getting ready to go to work, he was combing his hair after getting out of the shower when he found a raised purple lesion on his scalp. He said nothing to me, but when he came out of the bathroom, he seemed distracted. I thought maybe it was an intimacy thing. *Shrinks,* I thought, *you'd think they'd know better.* This seemed confirmed when later in the day and for the next few days he didn't return my calls.

I tried over and over again to think about what I might have said or done to give him offense. I figured that if he hadn't had a good time on the date, he would just say he didn't want to go out. But not refuse to answer my telephone calls. I didn't think that an issue with intimacy would cause this man to be rude and thoughtless, perhaps just difficult. Well, I was only 29.

Finally, I dropped by his office to see if he was OK. He took me outside and apologized for not calling, but then he told me about the lesion. I froze wide-eyed. He had had a biopsy to determine whether it was KS, and he would be getting it back that day or the next. I left his office feeling that I had just been handed my own diagnosis. *Not only did he have a lesion but it was a KS lesion,* I thought to myself. KS like Richard had. KS that would now pass somehow to me.

For the rest of the day I could concentrate on nothing else other than that he was going to get a call, like so many people I had met already, that was going to tell him he had KS. There was no HIV antibody test still. I couldn't go and get tested and find out if I was infected. I could only live with the knowledge that someone I had slept with may have been ill. No one from my sexual past had gotten sick, although frankly there had not been very many. Now I had slept with someone while he was ill, and he even discovered his condition in my own bathroom. *God.*

It was everything I could do to keep myself from calling him every ten minutes and asking if he had heard from the doctor. I watched my phone at home and at my office, willing it to ring with every fiber of my being. The span of time allowed my over-active mind to work in the most arcane ways. I am most singularly talented when it comes to this, and I opened up boxes of tragic possibilities to find all the other boxes inside, opening each one to some new tragedy. I would be diagnosed with KS. My family would suffer. I would have to quit my job. I could never go back home again, since it would put a black mark on my family. I wouldn't be able to get treatment any where other than New York. I would look like Richard. I had met the enemy, and he was me.

Finally the telephone rang. It was him.

"There is good news, and there is bad news."

I hate it when people say this. It drags things out unnecessarily, and it confuses my linear thought lines. I always make the same choice. I ask for the bad news so that the good news can undo some of the ill effect one feels from hearing the bad news, and one can walk away and say, "See, my day just got a little brighter." Taking the good news first, leaves it only to be ruined by the bad news. "Bad news," I said. "Give me the bad news."

"It is cancer," he said.

"Good news," I said, my heart in my throat.

"It's not KS—just plain old cancer."

"Thank God," I said. "The good news—just plain old cancer. I'm so happy for you."

The world had grown truly ironic.

We didn't see each other anymore. I think the strain of the situation was just a little too much for a first date. Now one might stop to think that having had this close call, it would have been prudent for me to have never slept with another man again. That would have been prudent. But it would not have been natural or even really possible. People are celibate for all sorts of good reasons, but fear isn't a good one. Fear isn't a good basis for any decision. That is one of the best lessons of this horrible epidemic.

## LEAVING THE MAINSTREAM WORLD BEHIND

"Riding a wave" is a California expression connected with surfing that I wouldn't become familiar with until later, but I knew what it meant. A wave appeared on my horizon, and I grabbed on to it. What began as a sort of philanthropic adventure by volunteering was rapidly becoming a consuming lifestyle. Perhaps it was the effect of seeing people die at a young age, but I was determined that I would make a startling move. And so in the spring of 1984 I left the investment firm. While I very much liked my job there, I found the circumstances under which I had to work to be increasingly oppressive. I believe that there may have been ample suspicion that I was gay. The oppressiveness may have been contrived to achieve the very result it did. I'll never know. Not long before I left the firm my office mate Richard overheard me in a telephone call where I was arranging to go see a client about getting his will done at a hospital. Richard said to me, "If you want to expose yourself to that shit, that's your business, but you have no call bringing it into the office." Even giving Richard the benefit of the doubt, it being 1984, I didn't have much patience with this attitude. I assured him that he and I weren't going to do anything in the office together that would result in my passing AIDS on to him. Still, it was a warning shot fired across my bow, and I suspected this attitude would only grow in intensity over time. I might be dead in a few years myself; I didn't want to die working for this firm. So I gave three weeks' notice, went computer and office-furniture shopping, and opened my own law practice.

In leaving the investment firm, I went from having a corner office in the Seagram building with a view that allowed me to see airline jets land at both airports to a charming little attic-like office on lower Madison Avenue with a view of sky and an occasional visit from a pigeon or two. The insecurity of it all and the uncertainty that lay behind my future income was terrifying and exhilarating. I cashed in some investments and borrowed $5,000 from my best friend. I sublet the office from a small firm of three gay attorneys. Eventually they took on a fourth, but I wanted to stay independent. Of those four, two have since died of AIDS and one died of a brain tumor that was not AIDS-related.

The practice was a successful enough start, helped out by many friends and my new office mates. However, six months into the practice Steve Gittleson, who had been working at Gay Men's Health Crisis as director of legal services, announced his intention to return to his own private practice, which he had put on hiatus while administering the new legal program. I was asked if I was interested in replacing him, but I wanted to give the new legal practice a chance, so I turned it down. Six months later the position was being offered again. The year of private practice had been an interesting experiment in my own doubtful courage, but it was not a passion for me. It became like any other job, except that I was my own boss. But the position at GMHC was something that was going to put me on the cutting edge of a new field of law. And it not only would be professionally satisfying in that respect but would be a position in which I would be very needed by the people who would be my clients, offering a feeling of emotional satisfaction at the same time. I grabbed the wave for all it was worth, and this time when the job was offered to me in the late spring of 1985 I took it. When I did, it was with the full consciousness that I was leaving the world of the Fortune 500 behind, giving up corner offices on Park Avenue and the potential for a nice salary and a real retirement plan (not a priority in the AIDS activist community) forever—no one rides a wave backward. While I had no qualms about this, it still had an impact. I was turning my back on everything my family and my legal training told me I had wanted. And some part of me did want it. Some part of me still wants it today. I often wonder what it would have been like if I had been able to stay there. Or for that matter what would it have even been like to be straight and not be a part of the nether world of gay men in the time of AIDS? I can't even imagine.

A few months before my arrival at GMHC, Rodger left his position as executive director. He had done quite an impossible job during his two years there and had positioned GMHC as the premier agency in the city dealing with people with AIDS, moved them into a smart set of offices from the dank basement in Chelsea (it seemed dank basements were to be the birthplaces of all AIDS organizations in those days in New York), and kept the agency afloat, raising money for what people said was an impossible cause. He was controversial, cutting edge, and "in your face" with the media and with city officials, who were learning from GMHC how to handle an urban health crisis.

After I accepted the new job I attended Rodger's going-away

party, held at the Café Bruxxels in the Village. It was an odd experience, the air being laced with some tension, given the change of administration from the colorful Rodger McFarlane to the more urbane and austere Richard Dunne. Larry Kramer, who was having his problems with GMHC, did not attend. Rodger was inexcusably late, a sign that he didn't really want to be there, and showed up with Brad Davis, who stayed only momentarily. Brad was appearing in Larry's off-Broadway production of *The Normal Heart*. He and I had met once or twice backstage, but each time he gave me only a short little nod or handshake.

I was more than excited to start this new job. But I was not without apprehension. I had never regarded myself as a particularly strong person before, and I knew this job was going to be difficult, but at the same time, it offered me an opportunity to fight my fear of the epidemic by facing it straight on—something I wasn't going to get by myself. In June 1985 I wrote in my diary, "Anyone observing me from the outside might think I'm bad in a crisis…. I'm still leading a normal life in a sea of madness. It is not the strong who survive at all—I've seen the strong come and go—it is the adaptable who survive." That is what it meant to me. When I began work at GMHC, Rock Hudson's diagnosis was not yet revealed, and most of America was still unaware of what was occurring in New York, San Francisco, and Los Angeles. I thought of it as the silent war, like when America was bombing Cambodia during the Nixon administration and no one knew anything about their tax dollars supporting such an event. AIDS was a war occurring in our midst and every day I rode the subway to work with people around me who as yet had little idea of what the AIDS epidemic meant. When they did encounter it, all hell would break loose, children being evicted from schools because they knew someone with AIDS and people losing their jobs because they were limp-wristed. Suddenly that was more than a mannerism; it meant contagion. All that was yet to come. AIDS was not a blip on any screen outside those cities and outside the people most affected.

GMHC was not a big corporation then. I was at first alone in my department. While later I was provided with a paid administrative assistant, in the beginning there was me, 600 clients, about 25 or 30 regular volunteers, and an IBM Selectric typewriter. The substance of the work was overwhelming. There was a backlog of hundreds of cases to face.

By that time my work with deathbed wills had become more routine, and once in this job I even became accustomed to doing what I referred to as my hospital rounds. I would start out in lower Manhattan, perhaps at Beekman Downtown, traveling up the east side to visit Cabrini, Bellevue, New York Hospital, Sloan Kettering, or Lenox Hill, then up to the Bronx to Metropolitan and down to Roosevelt with, of course, a stop off in Hell's Kitchen at St. Clare's. I got used to the challenge, although there were days that broke my heart when some young men would walk into my office for a will consultation. Oftentimes, the client would recite ordeals that sounded more like an arcane bar-exam question than it would a real-life human story.

"I don't know why I'm doing my will, anyway," he might say. "I don't really have much left. After my insurance dropped me, I had to pay for everything. I couldn't pay my bills, and I'm being dunned. I lost my job when I was diagnosed. My sister's husband won't let me see my nieces and nephews, and my parents have disowned me."

"Excuse me for a moment," I would say, wanting to take a break just to go out of my office for a private moment to marvel at the lengths some people would go to avoid contact with people who were infected. The stories were too ridiculous and cruel to be made up. Families torn apart, so-called Christian parents who would throw their own offspring out of the house because they were gay or ill or both. One life after another found its way into the office, disrupted, destroyed, and in the most utter pain.

Once one got used to the chaos, however, it became like any other crisis. After a while in the new job I got caught up with the caseload and even began to feel slightly ahead of things. I was a quiet young lawyer, working in a small office, barely getting the attention of anyone other than my volunteers and my clients and my new boss, a man named Richard Dunne, a stern and highly disciplined man who tolerated no bullshit and knew his mission well. He had been in the military, and that's how he ran the office.

The view from my new office was the corner of 18th Street and Eighth Avenue. It was a lively corner, and it was a great place to people-watch and see an occasional handsome man stroll by. This brought me almost as much opportunity for daydreaming as the view of both airports had at the investment firm. At least I could comfort myself with the fact that I still had a corner-office view, stark contrast though it was. And while the routine of what we had to do never really became too routine, crisis did become routine. I got better at interviewing clients in ways which were not threatening, and sometimes were empowering for them.

There were 17 other employees at GMHC. Richard was a consummate professional. He was the perfect candidate to take the agency to its next level, just as Rodger had been ideally suited in his talents for getting the impossible off the ground. Richard was set to institutionalize values that were professional and was determined in an agency nurtured on hysteria and reaction. Richard died not long after stepping down as executive director of the agency in 1990 or so. He died of PML, a disease so little known that there were only a few doctors in the world who had ever treated it. Tragically, it was a disease that robbed him of his motor skills to the point that walking across the street was a challenge. His speech was slurred. It was the height of indignity for a man who so cherished his own dignity.

But, as Richard wanted it, we did become more professional, even though at the same time, we were a close-knit family of sorts, working in a grassroots organization, dealing with people no one wanted to deal with—and all the time fearing that any day any one of us might be transformed from employee to client.

That happened a lot. Of those 17 other people who were working at the agency, I can think of only six of us who are alive today—Sandi Feinblum, Chuck Jones, Audrey Hassell, Mark Chataway, Barry Davidson, and me. My friend Bill Jones began work just after I did and went on to work for AIDS Project Los Angeles. With the two jobs, Bill was probably the one person overseeing the largest efforts at raising money for HIV. The others are all gone. Paul Carro was the accountant. He managed the books during a time when the agency went from having a budget of a few thousand dollars to several million, becoming its financial officer. Paul was young and sexy and when time permitted he had a great sense of humor. When he died a few years later he looked like a little old Italian man. He aged 40 years in the span of only two. At one point one of his lungs detached and had to be surgically reunited with his body.

Christopher was the Grace Kelly of gay men—cool, blond, and blue-eyed exterior covering what was surely a great fire, as Alfred Hitchcock said about the star princess. Christopher was the monitor of taste and decorum at the agency. It was Christopher who I took with me to shop for my tuxedo the night of the big joint benefit between ARC, GMHC, and AMF. Eventually he would leave the agency to take up a swanky position with Dunhill, but he later died in Virginia with his family.

Raymond Jacobs, an educator, led the first training I ever went to, and in a flamboyant style that was uniquely characteristic of him, he brought people together to talk about their fears and challenges in working with people with AIDS. Raymond would begin each training session by asking everyone in the room for the name of their favorite flower. Thereafter, we would be divided into groups based on that choice. Raymond was diagnosed with KS not long before I started working at GMHC (he was the one whose diagnosis Rodger had told me about just before our trip to Puerto Rico, sending the morale of the agency into a tailspin).

Diego was Puerto Rican, a social worker who was the director of client services. Before his death he had written a characteristically flamboyant and elaborate will that was typical of a true control queen. His will dictated that a party be held at the expense of his estate. It was a fabulous dinner and extravaganza on board a Circle Line boat that toured around the entire island of Manhattan with everyone drinking and laughing and dancing. It was quite an affair, managed by his best friend, Barry Davidson, one of my fellow survivors.

Later everyone working in an AIDS agency would almost expect as a matter of course that people among them would be prone to diagnosis and death. Raymond lived for a long time after his diagnosis but died in the '90s.

Audrey Hassell, another survivor, helped people hook into benefits programs, working with social security officers who were too afraid to even touch the application papers of a person with this disease. Audrey was an African-American heterosexual who understood what this disease meant back then and, more importantly, what it would mean in the future to people of color.

Another survivor, Sandi Feinblum, worked in client services in the starring role of concerned and serious lesbian. She was also someone you were glad was on your side.

And yet another, Mark Chataway, was the director of communications, trying to get AIDS and GMHC into the press as much as possible, which at the time was a daunting task. Today, Mark is an executive in a public-relations firm in London.

We all worked in our own worlds, all very different people who would have had very little to do with one another in real life. But as with any crisis, we were simply people who banded together, lifting the sandbags, handing them to the stranger next to us, taking little account of whether we really liked our co-worker. There wasn't much time for that sort of thing. We were distracted by our own needs, the needs of our clients, and our isolation from our own friends and families. But also, I think, by a vague perception that this was all too unbelievable to be really happening. In so many ways we became like family. We didn't choose our members, but even when we didn't like one another, we still loved one another with a fierce loyalty. And we were all very, very frightened.

Sometimes the experience reminds me of the murder mystery *Ten Little Indians,* by Agatha Christie. You had to wonder who would be next to go. We worked in the crisis, and every day seemed to be one, with no one on the outside really noticing what was going on. It all happened too fast to piece together. A horrible, contagious disease caused by something unknown came out of nowhere—just like that. It was like science fiction. People got diagnosed, went into the hospital, and died. Our receptionist died of a heart attack after his diagnosis while receiving treatment for pneumonia, but he was only in his 30s. Some of us often referred to it as a silent war, happening in the midst of everyday society, and while soldiers fought at the front lines, the rest of society stayed back, untouched at their borders. The war was even more remote than the one in Vietnam because at least the media had brought that war into everyone's living room. But the battle against AIDS got little attention, and the only living rooms it entered were those of people who had the disease, and the friends and family who stuck by them.

## THE MEDIA SUDDENLY DISCOVER AIDS

The French and the Americans had a long-standing dispute over who eventually discovered AIDS, or at least the virus that causes it. But the real discovery of AIDS in American did not occur in a lab; it occurred in the media. In 1985 an event occurred that grounded the health crisis in the minds of the American public. In fact, if you ask most Americans when the AIDS crisis began, they would probably say 1985. Then, something happened that changed the course of AIDS history, my job, my life, and the entire collective mind-set of America. Rock Hudson's AIDS diagnosis was made public. The impact of the announcement of Hudson's illness was no less than cataclysmic and in some ways miraculous at the way it transformed our little world at GMHC. AIDS jumped from the background of everyone's mind to the forefront, with no accompanying education. It was like yelling fire in the crowded movie theater called America. It was also the first inkling that when it came to AIDS, the emperor had no clothes. Surely at last the president would come out of his cocoon and make a statement about his friend Rock Hudson. He would say that this had gone on for long enough and that it was time to get down to the business of saving people's lives. After all, Rock was a fellow actor. But the president didn't do that; he merely maintained his judgmental silence, confirming our place out there on the edge.

The little office of GMHC, now located at 18th Street and Eighth Avenue in Chelsea, was besieged by the media, and Mark Chataway suddenly had a deluge of reporters to deal with. Camera crews, radio talk shows, newspapers, magazines, wire services—all focused on a little three-story building housing a restaurant, and on the top floors, GMHC. They could not get enough of us after virtually ignoring us for almost four years. Their understanding of the epidemic was ludicrous. They insisted on labeling people with AIDS as victims or patients, even though these very people explicitly made the point that they did not want to be called victims or patients because it detracted from their own struggle to not be treating AIDS as a death sentence. But the media wouldn't grant them even that shred of hope. "I don't get it," reporters would say time and time again. Yet not one of those same reporters would ever dare refer to an African-American as a Negro in print. Why? Black people had always been called Negro until they repudiated it as a slur to their self-esteem, and then no one called them Negro. Yet the media could not find it in their hearts to examine the issue of self-esteem for the person with AIDS. Why? Confounded by it at the time, I can only think now that it was easier for people who were well to think of people with AIDS as victims or patients because they had to.

I used to love to turn the tables on reporters interviewing me on some aspect of AIDS and ask them about whether they felt safe about their own sexual practices. They didn't like being drawn in by that. People didn't feel safe from AIDS but calling people with AIDS "victims" created a gulf of identity between "them" and "us." That, anyway, is the Senakian theory. As I've watched the media cover the issue, however, from the first mention of AIDS in *The New York Times* on page 27 in July 1981 through Rock Hudson to Magic Johnson to the gays-in-the-military issue to Brad Davis to Arthur Ashe to Greg Louganis, I sometimes think that if the modern media were covering the Emancipation Proclamation, there would be still slavery in America today. At any rate, in 1985 AIDS, like some dormant insect, emerged as a miracle of nature into the consciousness of the press and therefore America.

Suddenly AIDS was everywhere. AIDS in the workplace, AIDS in hospitals, AIDS in schools, AIDS in sports, AIDS on the subway. The topic of AIDS permeated America. Those scions of enlightenment, talk-radio hosts, found new fodder by the acre in this epidemic. The media are only reactive beasts at best, and their real ability to see the big picture is evident only when such a circumstance would coincide with really good ratings.

Those of us at GMHC were suddenly being asked to appear on all the talk shows. I was riding the talk-show circuit as if I had just published a best-seller or were promoting my latest film. In my off hours I could be seen at Macy's buying a stack of blue shirts because the camera crews seemed to get upset if you were wearing white. Besides, I looked better in blue. My mother's aunt telephoned my mother when I appeared on *Nightline* and said, "You'd better turn on the TV; your kid is on it," and then she hung up.

After the initial shock and news stories covering "our reaction" to the announcement came some initial if stumbling efforts at educating the public. It is a fact that in the course of the epidemic people do not change their belief system or level of concern about AIDS until they know someone who has it. To some degree Rock Hudson did that for people. America was shocked again when they saw him pose with Doris Day and later learned of his last-ditch efforts at getting treatment in Paris. For mainstream America, it was all a learning process—learning that AIDS existed, learning that it devastated beauty, learning that it killed. For those of us inside the AIDS beltway, there was some acknowledgment of the inevitable occurring but also, at least for me, some hopes were pinned to Hudson. The treatment he was flying to Paris to take was one of a long string of magic bullets. Even if they weren't billed as magic bullets, that was how they were interpreted. People wanted so badly to believe in something. With Hudson, I hoped they wouldn't let him die. When he flew to Paris I could imagine that the promising new treatment he sought, HPA-23, might take hold and that he would serve as a catalyst for its delivery to all those now suffering and avoiding what was going to come. Of course, it didn't happen that way.

But much of the early press attention was on The Kiss. The Kiss was a scene everyone was recalling from the night-time soap opera *Dynasty,* where Rock Hudson was seen passionately kissing Linda Evans. Later it would be AIDS on the basketball court with Magic Johnson. Could other players get it? For other actors, when Brad Davis died the question was, Could they have contracted it by working with him? It was the same with boxers in the ring or players on the football field. Could the other divers get AIDS from Greg Louganis?

The media attention was frenzied. Those of us who were working with people with AIDS, who had lost friends, were resentful. After all, he wasn't the first person to be diagnosed. Other people went before him. Weren't their stories important too? It was a sentiment that would be echoed in 1991, when Magic Johnson's announcement made an even bigger impact. Still, the announcement was like rain in the desert. Now everyone thought about AIDS, even if their thoughts were wild and panicked.

America was so afraid. People were understandably perceiving only the danger. They saw only that AIDS was contagious and fatal. The media failed miserably in conveying the important aspects of AIDS. The media could not convey the AIDS epidemic because it was too complex for them to understand and they were too busy to take the time to try. It shook my faith in the media's ability to understand the truth, a faith that had been built on a foundation of Watergate, when the media reigned supreme as our national conscience.

When Rock Hudson died, discrimination cases seemed to suddenly proliferate. People only knew that AIDS=Fatal=Fear. The climate provided a virtual cultured petri dish for discrimination. Cases of discrimination, which before had come into the office on the order of one per week, mushroomed to one per day. People saw The Kiss in the context of their own lives. Something new began to happen with more frequency, however. The circle of discrimination that had formed around the newly diagnosed now widened to encompass people who for one reason or another were perceived to have AIDS. It might be a perceived effeminacy or a persistent cough or a bruise that wouldn't go away. Guilt by association was a common occurrence. One woman who came to my office had lost her fiancé to AIDS. She missed a few days of work, and when she returned she confided in a friend what had happened. This friend then apparently informed management. The following day an armed security guard escorted the woman from the premises and asked her not to come back until she could produce a negative HIV antibody test. Children were kicked out of school in Westchester and Queens, not because they had HIV but because they either had a family member with HIV or merely knew someone with AIDS.

The media took a typical approach, pitting one extreme

against another, looking for the ends of both extremes in the hope that people discern the truth somewhere in the middle and in the further hope that the drama of the situation would help ratings. But in the middle of truth and myth, they themselves were afraid. I can recall a crew coming to the office one day for a comment on some new aspect of AIDS, wanting me to come down to the street for an interview. I leaned out my window and invited them up to my office. They said they'd rather do the interview in the street. As it turned out, the crew got hazard pay for coming into my office, the kind of pay they got for accompanying a SWAT team or going into a war zone. Hazard pay to talk to little old me. Another of my colleagues had had a lapel microphone snipped off his lapel with scissors because the technician was afraid to take it back.

At this time I also learned a real lesson about radio call-in shows. Don't do them. At least it is important to check out the show's background first to make sure you don't get caught in one of those lose-lose situations. One radio call-in guy was screened by the communications director of GMHC, and I agreed to do the show by telephone. He sounded very reasonable and pleasant on the telephone, but when we got on the air he became a ranting, hostile demagogue. "So," he said on the air, "it's true that most gays practice anal intercourse, isn't it, and that's how it's spread. Right? So in a few years you'll all be dead anyway, so why should we try to find a cure for AIDS? I mean you're all gonna die anyway?" I discontinued participation by hanging up.

Nevertheless, I went on the talk-show rounds, local and national. At first I wanted everything to be taped, naively assuming that if I said anything stupid, they would edit it out. Quite the opposite was actually true. One morning I was called by news media to the steps of the cathedral on Fifth Avenue in New York. The issue was housing and people with AIDS. Interviewing Cardinal O'Connor on one end of the steps, the cameras rushed over to my end to interview me. It was a long and mostly pointless interview. In the end what ran was a sound byte in which, with my defenses down, I said something glib and sarcastic rather than objective and substantive. The same could be said for the cardinal. If you had watched the news that night, you wouldn't have learned anything about AIDS or the cardinal or myself; you would have seen two opposing viewpoints poorly expressed. You would not have learned anything about AIDS, you would have only seen a little drama. In this sense, news, especially local television news efforts, become less a news broadcast and more of a field of scant entertainment at best.

In no time I gained my street smarts to learn that I preferred live so that no one could control what I said. Some reporters would want to come to my home, but I wouldn't allow anyone inside, because I felt it was too intrusive. Since I was listed in the telephone book, I sometimes got hate mail and death threats during this time, especially when I would appear on television with respect to a discrimination matter. That was intrusive enough.

But my favorite media event occurred not long after the Rock Hudson diagnosis. As I've noted, with the sudden awareness of AIDS and its dangers coupled with really very little knowledge, discrimination became sort of rampant and in some respects hysterical. At one point Mayor Koch administration announced that a nursing home in Queens would be made into an AIDS residence. One of the lessons learned early on in the epidemic is that when you do this sort of thing you do advance work in the neighborhood and get everyone on a somewhat level playing field of knowledge about AIDS before you make announcements. This was an oversight. The people in this section of Queens did not want the Neponsit Nursing Home turned into the sort of place that attended to AIDS patients. Never mind the fact that we were talking about AIDS and that we knew many others who were infected with HTLV-III, as it was then called, rode the subway with us every morning. Once a person had "AIDS," he crossed a line into the untouchable realm. It was known that some people had what was called ARC, which stood for AIDS-related complex, meaning that you were infected and maybe sick but you didn't have AIDS. There was a growing understanding that people were infected without yet being sick. However, people generally did not understand the distinction between AIDS and infection with the virus. On the one hand, they were all "AIDS" people, but it didn't seem to occur to members of the general public or the media that each day almost each New Yorker was in all likelihood near or with someone who was infected. They weren't afraid of what they didn't know, but once they knew you had AIDS, they knew to be afraid.

A local talk show was going to cover the debate and protest, which had been eating up the headlines of the past few days. They wanted to have on camera a PWA, myself, and some people from Queens who were protesting the decision. They were also having Harold Jaffe from the Centers for Disease Control.

The afternoon of the show, which was a live format, the network affiliate called. It was the show's producer who wanted to say that their PWA had gotten sick and could I recommend someone.

"Sure," I said. "A friend of mine and a client of ours, David Summers, just passed by my door and stuck his head in to say hello. He is media-experienced and articulate, and he would be great. I'll grab him and see if he wants to do it, and I'll bring him with me."

There was no answer on the other end.

"That's OK, we'll send a crew out to him and have him on remote. The people from Queens are going to be on remote too."

"Well, you don't need to bother," I said. "I can bring him with me. It's no trouble, especially since you're sending a car for me anyway."

"No," she said kind of stubbornly, "we'd rather do the remote."

"Why?" Another long pause. I still don't get it.

"Well, look, I have to tell you; our crew doesn't want a PWA in the studio."

"You're kidding me."

"No, so we'll just send out the remote," she said.

"No," I said. "I'll be bringing him with me."

"I can't do that," she said.

"Well, then, I'll tell you what. It is 1:20 and we go on at 5. Then this means you have 20 minutes of dead airtime this afternoon, because if he doesn't go on with me, I don't do the show."

"You can't do that."

"I think I can."

"But you promised."

"I know. I'm taking it back," I said.

"I want to talk to Lori Behrman," she said. Lori Behrman had taken the place of Mark Chataway as communications director when he left the agency.

"OK," I said.

A few minutes later Lori came into my office. She wasn't terribly happy with me, which concerned me because we had become (and still are) good friends. But I was taking a stand that was firm—I was beginning to discover my own sense of activism. Lori saw that I was not only resolute but also that it was the right thing to do even though her professional instincts told her that we shouldn't offend the media. But with the Rock Hudson diagnosis, the tables had turned. It used to be the rule that we needed the media we needed to appease them to get our message out. Now it was a different ball game; they needed us.

Over the course of the afternoon there were many phone calls back and forth. Finally, the affiliate called to say that if staff walked off the set, then management would step in and run the cameras. In the late afternoon a car came and picked up David and me, and we were met at the newsroom door by the show's producer. We stood outside and she said, "Look, I don't know what's going to happen in there, but I think this turned out all right."

We walked into the newsroom, which was one of those long, long expanses with a low drop ceiling and fluorescent lighting with a ramble of tossed-around desks and computer terminals. Everyone looked up at us and it got kind of quiet. David looked relaxed and tanned and fit and healthy. He was also very handsome. I, on the other hand, didn't look so hot and was frankly pale and tired. I think everyone thought I was the PWA.

We sat in the green room and tried to make small talk without much success, but it wasn't long before we had to walk onto the set of the show. We went through a large door, and the set was off in the distance with a crowd of people between us and the set. Ladders were propped up to banks of lights overhead. Again the room got eerily quiet. David and I stood there and looked out at the silhouettes of people, though we really couldn't see any faces. I looked at David and reached over and took him by the hand. We walked into the crowd, which parted as if we were Norma Desmond herself. We got up to the stage, and no one really moved. A little man, the kind who looked like he'd been working sound since television began, came up and pinned a lapel mike on David. David said, "Thanks," and the man patted David's shoulder. It was like some signal to the rest of the crew, and in a few minutes we were on the stage and in our seats. As I sat down, the light above me exploded. I started and again grabbed David Summers's hand.

"I thought someone shot me," I said honestly.

"That's OK," he said. "I thought someone shot you too." We laughed hard as the show came in off its commercial break, and we were on without incident, except TV viewers had to wonder why we were grinning from ear to ear.

In the end most reporters were not thoughtful, especially those on a local level who seemed not only disinterested in anything of substance in the stories they covered but determined to avoid it at all costs. Television reporters are under particular pressure to get the sound byte they need and to run to the next talking head they can find to get another. Time for researching and understanding the issue is nonexistent. I can recall sitting in my office trying to explain the concept of an HIV antibody test to a local female reporter. I could not get her to come to grips with the fact that the test was not really an "AIDS test," as the media had dubbed it, but rather a test for an antibody to the virus believed to cause AIDS. In those days it was uncertain what that meant. It could mean that you had been exposed but would never develop AIDS. I tried four different times in four different ways to explain it. Lori Behrman stood in the corner of my office. Lori and I could exchange a lot of words in a glance. Her eyes kept telling me to try again. Finally, her eyes rolled down to the floor as if to say, *I can't believe she doesn't get it.* I gave up. The reporter never understood.

It is not fair to generalize. One very hot and humid day in the summer of 1985 a reporter came to my home to interview me about children in school with AIDS. The school year was just beginning, and this was a drama unfolding in Queens. It seemed like these cases all took place in Queens. I did the interview in the hallway of my building, sticking to my desire not to have reporters in my home. It was hot and humid and sticky, and the interview went badly. I did not feel good about my responses. The reporter was taller than me by a head, which I found intimidating when he kept putting his face down to mine while he seemed accusatory in the nature of his questioning. He was truly in my face on the issue, interrupting me and inserting himself into the interview. After it was over I went inside and took off my damp shirt and tie and khakis and put on a pair of shorts and tank top. The telephone rang, and it was the reporter. He wanted to reshoot the second half of the interview because he felt he had been unfair, biased by the fact that he had two children in school himself, and he confessed to feeling emotional about the issue. He admitted the interview was highly biased. I looked at my damp clothes, now wrinkled on the floor, and agreed to reshoot the second half.

## TAKING A BATH

Not all reporters were thoughtless, particularly on the national level. But local media is nothing less than a waste of air space. There was a local talk show that I did a few times during 1985 in New York. One of the shows pitted me in debate against the Republican candidate for mayor, Diane McGrath. She was a pleasant woman to talk to. I know because we were both early and shut into the green room and we had a pleasant chat. I felt kind of sorry for her and wondered where the Republican Party had found her. She had no chance of beating Ed Koch, and everyone knew it. On some level she knew it too. She seemed to be some sacrificial lamb that the Republicans were putting up for slaughter, and I could only hope that she was going through with this humiliation for the purpose of getting some other office later down the road from grateful party officials. She deserved it.

She seemed to have a lot of trouble finding some municipal issues around which to build a platform for her campaign. That, as it turns out, is always a dangerous thing for public health policy and AIDS. Because whenever politicians have nothing that they can otherwise do, they are naturally drawn to AIDS, emitting a smoke screen that makes it look like they are doing something about a problem when in fact they are doing nothing at all or even making the situation worse.

Diane McGrath's views represented the school of thought that says it is good to punish people with the virus; in stigmatizing them you make it look like you are doing something about the epidemic. In a politically bankrupt position she had little choice but to look to AIDS to solve her problems. Otherwise, she would have found it hard to get a mention in the papers. Therefore, she embarked on a campaign to close the gay bathhouses in New York City to stop the spread of AIDS.

My boss, Richard Dunne, was going on vacation. Before leaving he asked me to handle a televised debate for him on the subject of bathhouse closure and to "make mincemeat out of her." There was a slight problem in this for me. I had never been to a gay bathhouse. I did not have negative feelings about people who went to them; I just felt that they were not something that appealed to me. They signified a use of another person that was not a way in which I wanted to behave toward others, nor was it how I wanted to be treated. But I very much recognized that that was my own decision about me and my life. I did not want others to make their decisions based on my feelings. People need to base their conduct on their own feelings. McGrath's position was that the bathhouses contributed to AIDS because sex goes on there. I had to take her word for that, since I had no experience of it.

Today the public health arguments that run counter to her position are apparent. They were not so apparent to me in 1985. So I studied Diane McGrath. Out of a meager 14 articles that had appeared about her in *The New York Times*, 11 of them were about her position on gay bathhouses. I could think of millions of problems that were facing the city of New York in 1985, and the gay bathhouses weren't among the first million. I asked several people I knew about the issue.

I regarded the bathhouse as a symbol of the generation of gay men who came before me, the men and women who were involved in the Stonewall riots of 1969, when police tried to raid a gay bar and found that they met with some intense and riotous opposition. Stonewall was an event that had commanded the respect of all gay and lesbian people. It was the reaction of people who were tired of being pushed to the side and despised by society. They were people who—more than being tired of being despised—were tired of their own closets. Gay bathhouses are after all only an expression of the reality of sexual constraint imposed on gay people by a straight society.

Once a reporter asked me why gay men liked to go to bathhouses and have sex with so many other men. I asked him to pretend for a moment that when he grew up, instead of a mom and dad, he had two moms or two dads. Pretend further, I said, that you grew up knowing that you were different from your two moms or your two dads and that in fact the entire world seemed gay to you. You grow up knowing you are different because you know you like girls, I said. You have a tendency to be masculine as a child, drawing the worried attention of your parents and making you a target at school with all the other little boys and girls. You are labeled even by your teachers as being "straight." Names like "breeder" are thrown out at you during junior high school, and in high school you often are beaten up because people suspect you of being a heterosexual. You learn to hide your heterosexuality and you date other boys, even though you lie in bed at night wondering what it would be like to have sex with a woman and feeling ashamed about it in the morning. Every commercial, every movie, every television you see your entire life is of gay people. Even *The New York Times* refuses to print the word "straight" in its pages, preferring "heterosexual" instead. Your family speaks sometimes in hushed tones about an errant uncle or aunt or cousin who is "different," and you know inherently that you are different in the same way. You occasionally hear stories or read items in the newspapers about straight people whose children are awarded custody to a gay couple or taken away by a gay parent because heterosexuals are considered to be unsuitable parents. You grow up imagining a world where you can be accepted. You grow up knowing that people shun you and that if you fall in love with some nice girl, the best you can hope for is that you can lead concealed lives together in privacy. People tell you that they don't mind what you do in private, as long as you don't flaunt your heterosexuality in public and that you must come to regard statements like that as open-minded. In fact, the law has so little respect for you and your relationships that not only can you never marry the person you love but in most states in the United States the act of sex with the person you love is a criminal offense. Finally, imagine that you are finally able to move to the big city, where there is a higher level of acceptance by people of who and what you are and that there are places where you can go and have all the sex you were told you could never have. Imagine that there are roomfuls of beautiful women who want you too. Imagine that you are told you can never get married. Years of repressing yourself and feeling ashamed of yourself for being who you are melt away with the opportunity.

Given that, I would finally ask the reporter, would you go to that bath house and would you have a good time if you knew you would never be married and that you weren't encouraged to have relationships legally sanctioned in any way? Or would you go without sex?

"I would go to the bathhouses," he said, decidedly. I smiled.

I believe that men in the Stonewall generation held onto the bathhouses very emotionally as a symbol of their liberation. Sexual relations, I believe, were an answer to the appetites denied so strongly growing up. Later generations, of course, go to bathhouses. Sexual liberation still occurs despite AIDS. But to the Stonewall generation, the bathhouses belong.

Because I had never been to one and had been pretty conservative when it came to sex, I was greatly uncomfortable about engaging in a live televised debate with a mayoral candidate on an issue that was very complicated and virtually impossible to convey in a sound byte. Her position was very simple and very clear: AIDS is spread by sex; sex occurs in bathhouses among gay men on a large scale; if you close gay bathhouses, there will be less AIDS. It sounded to me like it made sense.

I was no big fan of Ed Koch. Mayor Koch was, however, a good politician. Diane McGrath was grasping at any straw possible to get attention. I couldn't really blame her, except that her attempt was very much at the expense of the public by misleading them about AIDS. It was also an approach that was aimed at gay men, an easy target. In fact, if she wanted to make AIDS a campaign issue, the mayor was vulnerable. His first AIDS commission had no authority, no mandate, no budget, and therefore no point. While that would have been a legitimate mode of attack for her; it lacked the emotional appeal and target potential offered by the stigmatized role of gay men and gay sex.

However, before we went on the air I was able to overcome my discomfort about the debate after talking to a few people, most notably Rodger McFarlane. He has an uncanny ability to sense the most vulnerable point in any opposition and open it up without mercy. He also recognizes bullshit better than anyone I know. He helped me to see the bathhouse controversy for what it was, not in terms of sex but in terms of public health. As a public-health issue, closing bathhouses did not seem to make a tremendous amount of sense.

First of all, organizations like GMHC were reaching out to people who went to bathhouses with information about safer sex practices. If we closed the bathhouses, we lost our connection to them. A large number of men who use the bathhouses were not gay-identified men but men with families from outer New York City regions who would never identify as being gay even though they had sex with men. Close the bathhouses, and we would be cut off from them.

Sex did not cause AIDS, the conventional wisdom dictated. *Unsafe* sex caused AIDS. AIDS was not something that belonged to risk groups; it belonged to risky behavior. The most important way to combat the epidemic was not to tell people that they cannot have sex but to inform them how they can have sex safely. People have sex all the time. Telling them not to have sex, whether as a mayor or a cardinal, is not going to keep them from having sex. *Not* telling people how to have safer sex is going to kill people. I could never reconcile in my mind the position of the church to withhold condoms and safer-sex messages from teens while at the same time being vehemently opposed to abortion. Killing on the one hand comes easy; killing on the other does not. However, today there are new schools of thought that say that the unbridled, promiscuous sexual culture of gay men in fact did create catalytic conditions for an epidemic in gay America. That may be true today—hindsight is a wonderful thing—but back then it wasn't even culturally possible for that argument to be viably debated. As I've said before, we thought the world was flat, now we know it was round. In terms of the arguments made today that public-sex environments should be closed because they spread HIV, I cannot say I'm convinced that the issue is as black and white as some would have us believe. The polarization of viewpoints makes good copy but not good public health. None of that was clear to me heading into the debate. I had to consider my points as I knew them then.

Secondly, as was scientifically known by then, people getting AIDS had been infected at least several years before. Closing the bathhouses was the proverbial closing of the barn door long after the horse was gone.

So I went into the 20-minute live television debate against Diane McGrath armed to the teeth with information, talking incessantly, barely giving McGrath an opportunity. It was rude but effective. I made my public-health points, and I also laid out her record in the press on being all about bathhouses. I said it was the symptom of a candidate without a platform and that the voters of this city deserved better than this. I did as Richard requested I do. I made short work of her. Afterward she told me that I had espoused a lot of hype. "That," I replied, "is the pot calling the kettle black." Not a particularly original reply but apt nonetheless.

The media interest in AIDS continued to pick up steam. In May 1985 I published my first piece, an op-ed for *The New York Times* on HIV testing by insurance companies. Fearful of the potential loss of millions of dollars in the face of an epidemic, insurers had also embarked on an insidious warpath with the ferocity of Sherman attacking Atlanta, not against AIDS but against people with AIDS. The HIV antibody test was being used behind people's backs without consent or knowledge of the person being tested to screen people out from the insurance pools. Companies, in effect, were engaged in a number of practices that were causing people to be discriminated against on a massive scale. The consequences to public health were potentially devastating.

When the AIDS epidemic wasn't paid much attention by mainstream America and the media, insurance companies stood up and took note. In fairness, the potential liability to them if there were an uncontrollable epidemic is considerable. But also in fairness the business they are in is all about risk and their willingness to wager on certain events happening or not. Their job is to minimize their risk, take in premiums, invest in real estate, and pay their stockholders. But the AIDS epidemic and with it the test for HIV antibodies changed all this considerably. Health insurers found ways to drop people from their policies, leaving them to the mercies of the public health system. Later some insurers sought to minimize their liability by capping their insurance polices, stating that they would only cover, for example,

$5,000 over the course of a lifetime for conditions related to AIDS. Although the policy would cover up to $1 million for any other catastrophic illness. But perhaps the most insidious and far-reaching practices came with the advent of the HIV antibody test, when insurers would test people for HIV antibodies without their consent or knowledge. This would in turn brand the person tested as an uninsurable, a 20th-century American version of an untouchable in the eyes of insurance companies. In the face of AIDS the meaning of having insurance diminished it began to mean less and less, which has an impact far beyond people with HIV.

I published my first article about this, for *The New York Times* opinion page, which was titled "Ban the HIV Test." In the article I called the HIV test the Gold Star of the 1980s, serving only as a marker for discrimination. The antidefamation league called, furious that I would make an analogy between Judaism and AIDS. But like it or not, that is all the HIV test was then, except to signal to the individual infected that he should change his sex or needle-sharing practices. There was nothing that could be done to help people with AIDS, so testing was of little consequence to anyone but medical curiosity and subsequently insurers.

By allowing insurers to test, a dangerous precedent for testing was set for the future. As genetic science advances and we are able to screen people for a particular genetic proclivity to cancer or Alzheimer's or obesity, and we treat those test results vis-à-vis insurance companies in the same way that we have treated HIV, then insurance companies will be insuring only the healthy elite, while most of the public is left without insurance, except that provided by government. Fewer and fewer people will be able to buy insurance. By their own practices, I wrote, like greedy exploiters of natural resources, insurance companies will become obsolete.

Publishing that article was thrilling. I remember the day it came out; I went and bought about ten copies of the *Times*. Tom Wicker also had a column that day. I was so proud that my article was on the same page with Tom Wicker's. I imagined all kinds of New Yorkers waking up and drinking their coffee and reading my column. It was an exhilarating thought; the mayor, Jacqueline Onassis, some old boyfriend who dumped me. In my imagination that morning they were all reading it, pushing out a lower lip, and saying "not bad" to themselves. I didn't even want to cash the check from the *Times*; I wanted to save it always. But times being what they were, I cashed it. My sentimentality apparently has its price. It was $150.

## DOING WHAT I THOUGHT
## I COULD NEVER DO

I have always been insecure about my self-image. I have always felt that there was something wrong with me—that I was fat or too tall or too short. It really wouldn't ever matter what characteristic about myself would be the focus; one day I could be too fat, the next too thin. It was an issue for therapy, and after my experience with Chuck the Therapist, I began seeing someone, Jim Christon, a gay man with whom I was socially acquainted.

Jim was a good therapist, the kind who doesn't intrude himself into your therapy. He would ask questions but never provide answers. Rather his questions were of a nature that allowed you to discover the answers yourself. Early in our sessions, which went on for two years, I had a dream that so embarrassed me, I resolutely decided that I would not tell Jim. Within four minutes of our next session, I had told him everything.

I dreamed that I was pregnant. I have always wanted children and am especially good with infants. In the dream I was telling good friends that I was going to have a child. Progressively in the dream my naked belly grew larger and larger, and I ran my hands over it with pride while people marveled at the miracle of it. Also the bigger it got, the happier I became. I woke up smiling.

I thought this dream was one of the biggest compromises of my masculinity that I could imagine. I explained it to Jim, utterly mortified. He sat there in his usual stoic mode and looked at me for a moment.

"Why were you so happy in this dream?" he asked.

I thought it a stupid question. I felt like he hadn't been listening to me. I had always told him I liked children. I made the point again in case he had forgotten and told him that I was happy to be having a child, deliriously happy. Then I talked about some other aspects of the dream, or things I would remember suddenly.

"What made you so happy in the dream?" he asked again.

I thought Jim was having a bad day or not into the therapy session. I repeated everything for him again. Then he asked me what had been going on in my life lately. I told him that I had published a piece in the *Times* and that I had been on some talk shows and newscasts and that I was busy at work and that I was accepting several speaking engagement offers. A lot of things were happening that were very exciting for me. Near the end of the session, he asked me again why I was so happy in the dream.

I was exasperated with him. "Because," I said, "I was happy because I was having a child. I like children. Having children was something I always thought would be denied me because I was gay. I was happy because it was like I was thumbing my nose at the world and at fate and at all circumstances that had worked against me."

Then I blurted out, "I was happy because I was doing something that I always wanted to do but that I never thought I could do!"

I felt as dumb as dirt when I said that. Everything clicked into place. All the things in my life at that time—the writing, the publishing, television—these were all things that I had always wanted to do but never thought I could do. This included the conquering of so many of my own worst fears. It included being next to the bed of a dying person, facing off with mortality. I was happy because I was doing things I never thought I could do before. The meaning behind giving birth to all this was suddenly so clear and obvious. Now that sounds as though I was not terribly insightful, and perhaps I wasn't. But I found that the therapy session about that dream to be one of the most groundbreaking events of my life. I realized it was what was so cutting edge about squaring off with the epidemic; it constantly put you in the position of having to do things you never thought you could do before even if sometimes they were things you never wanted to do in the first place.

I don't want to even hint that the reason people started doing AIDS work had anything to do with the idea of self-empowerment, at least not consciously. But there is little doubt that being attracted to AIDS work brought with it more than a sense of altruism or fulfilling a need to be needed or a sense of duty to one's people; it also involved control.

By working in AIDS, I felt on some level that I was doing the only thing I could to control the madness around me. I could not stop friends from dying, people from suffering, or myself from getting AIDS. I could only control my environment within the context of the epidemic to the best of my ability, and if I did that, then I would be leading a better life. If I didn't, then I was truly going to be leading a life of pure fear. In that sense I really would become an "AIDS victim."

None of that was even remotely apparent to me then. The dream did not unlock some great analytical ability in me to suddenly realize this in 1985. But now I can more clearly see that one of the things that kept me involved in the epidemic was not wanting to lose that sense of empowerment, that sense of control, and the sublime feeling I got from knowing I was still doing things I would never have thought I could do. Each day I still uncover my ghosts who haunt me and my demons who can come in the night. If I ever stopped, how would I fight the demons?

Thinking back to those early days at GMHC, I am struck by the contrast with consciousness of AIDS today. That office over a restaurant on a busy Manhattan corner was a thousand years ago, hundreds of lifetimes ago. Richard Dunne, Paul Carro, Christopher, Diego Lopez, Raymond are all dead. Barry, Sandi, Audrey, Chuck, Mark Chataway, and I are alive. It had been such a long way to come, from disinfecting that glass that Paul drank from in my apartment in 1983 to being in bed with dying PWAs in 1984 to debating mayoral candidates on television in 1985. By midyear 1985 I felt that I had come just about as far as I could, and I doubted that there was much more I could learn or adapt to. Now it was just a matter of carrying on and waiting and wondering if I would live to see the end of this epidemic.

When I began my new position at GMHC in May I found that I was backlogged with several hundred cases of clients who had not yet gotten services, and each day more called. One day as I was sifting through and trying to organize and prioritize all the backlogged cases, a telephone call was from a man who was an actor-model-waiter. He said he had been fired from the very trendy restaurant where he worked in Manhattan because he had AIDS. I asked him what opportunistic infections he had had. He told me that it began with a bad case of shingles (herpes zoster), which is often the beginning sign of a compromised immune system. But the discharge from employment came, he said, when he had developed KS. I asked him if he had any lesions on his face, and he told me that one was beginning. I looked around my office for a clue as to what I could do for him. A waiter with KS, I thought to myself, some great discrimination case. I could picture Richard's face every time I saw anyone with a KS lesion—and every night before I went to sleep. I took a deep breath and, choosing my words carefully, I explained to him that I was alone and in the midst of a significant backlog and that I wouldn't be able to represent him at the time. I referred him to the city commission for human rights, where he would find help and where they would also advocate for him. It was a dodge, but I knew that they would help him and, given the number of cases I had already, I didn't think I could spend time and effort chasing after what might be a hard-won victory.

He tried to get me to change my mind, but I had to hold firm. I didn't think this was a case I could handle, and, what's more, it intimidated me. I tried to explain it to him.

He became angry and hung up on me. His name was Joe. He was going to be my spouse.

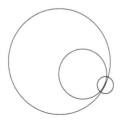

P A R T   T W O

J O E

*"I opened to my beloved;*
*but my beloved had withdrawn himself,*
*and was gone:*
*my soul failed when he spake:*
*I sought him, but I could not find him:*
*I called him but he gave me no answer."*

~SONG OF SOLOMON, CHAPTER 5, VERSE 6~

# Chapter 6: Late 1985

There was no way of knowing it that day on the telephone when the angry young waiter hung up on me, but if I had but the merest clue as to who he was, I would have begged to represent him. For many years there was a man I would see around town who I thought to be one of the most handsome and sensual men I had ever seen in my life. I had always wanted to talk to him. I did not know who he was. I had never known his name. But he was the waiter who had just hung up on me. With the clock of Joe's life ticking away, fate smiled upon me and my hopeless years of yearning and introduced us that day, though not on the best terms. And with that introduction began another clock, a span of time into which we would have to cram a lifetime of happiness and living. While I wouldn't give him my help that day, in the not too distant future there was nothing I would not have done to make him happy.

It is best that I be clear and direct on this point, for I think that simplicity is often the most poignant means of delivering a heartfelt sentiment. I loved Joe. Profoundly. With everything I had. Loving him was not like loving anything or anyone else in my life, though I suppose it is not an entirely fair proposition to compare the love of a lover with anything else; it is too much set apart. This was not a feeling that I had expected would necessarily come along in my lifetime, but I knew that if it did, I would count myself among one of the luckiest people on earth. I cannot say that I knew precisely what that love would feel like when it presented itself to me, but I was never without faith that when it did come, I would know it as readily as I would an old friend. I knew that as surely as I knew where my next breath came from. And when I finally did meet Joe, I knew what I felt was exactly what I had waited for all my life, and whether it lasted five minutes or 500 years I was happy and grateful for it. And I suspect just as surely that now that it has gone, I will never feel it again. Now it is a memory that I call to mind only infrequently, because, like the sun during an eclipse, I believe that staring at it too directly could cause me damage. Still, I count myself lucky to have seen it come and go just once. For me, loving Joseph was forging myth into being—writing the poem of perfection—and no act in my life will ever match it. I shall always be glad that for a while it was mine.

I can honestly say that as I begin to write this I get chills. Though I am trying my hardest to convey it, no one will ever truly know what those early days of the epidemic were like for me. Even now there must be some natural safety mechanism that automatically triggers, causing some of those memories to slip away in some unknown part of my consciousness like bits of an old movie. But when I think hard about Joseph, a sense of what they were comes back to me as easily as picking up a child's bottled snow scene that I can shake up and bring a flurry to a familiar setting, making it happen all over again. I can still smell his hair, his skin, and for a moment, I can look into his eyes. I can remember what it all was like for me in this respect with a startling clarity, but I don't know that anyone else will ever really know, no matter how hard I try to explain it.

I suppose that is the existential truth for us all—we are all alone and no one else in the universe quite knows what each of us goes through. I know for me that is sometimes a particularly lonely realization. This is especially true when it is something that has made me either terribly happy or woefully sad, and with Joseph both extremes are true. And so I would want you to know about Joe more than anything else because I think my story is mostly about love and happiness in the midst of so much chaos. And whatever my experience has been and whatever it will be, I will always remain a romantic. I think too that it says something very important about the history of this epidemic and the people it took and what happened to the people who are left. I want to tell about it because it is about death and about survival.

The first time I had ever seen him was sometime in the 1970s in Manhattan. That was such a different time, like the roaring '20s before the stock market crash and the Great Depression, which followed. I have always held the phrase *sexual revolution* in low regard, a mass-media-produced term that was supposed to characterize very individual experiences. But in the post-Stonewall era, sex between men was something that was more accepted and practiced more openly. People who disdain it are so unrealistic. They seem to feel that because gay men are disapproved of, then sex between them should not occur. But suffice it to say that post-Stonewall, people accepted their own identities with more abandon than before.

Joe had no identity for me other than being someone who

I thought was the most handsome man I had ever seen. And he was part of a world I did not fully comprehend nor which I could have naturally stepped into—a world of Studio 54, the Saint, and the kind of people who posed with sculpted bodies in magazine ads. They were people who seemed to all know each other, all with other handsome and beautiful friends. Where they didn't have friends, they could make them easily. They were people who defined the 1970s. They were comfortable with themselves, their sexuality, and sex itself. I on the other hand seem perpetually perplexed by all three, viewing them as mysteries that must be analyzed and if possible solved.

It was a weekend night, and I was in a bar called Uncle Charlie's in the Village having a beer. Uncle Charlie's was what we called an "S&M" bar. That doesn't stand for *sadomasochism;* it stands for *standing and modeling,* a pastime in which the patrons of the place were most frequently engaged. There wasn't much conversation, just standing around, drinking beer, posing, and throwing around as much attitude as possible.

Years later whenever I returned to New York I could still walk past there and glance in the window and see Joe as I did that one night years ago. He really knew S&M well. It worked for me. He had the type of appeal for me that can only be described as thunderstruck. That may sound corny now, but it was real. There are a lot of things that bring dead clichés to life. Falling in love is one of them.

He had a particular and unique kind of beauty. There was a rare quality to his smile, which caused deep lines to appear on both sides of a full and sensual mouth, exposing a beautiful set of teeth, for which, being an actor-model-waiter, he had paid a dentist good money. His mouth looked as if he weren't careful, he could swallow you while it kissed you. His eyes were large and would have been too close together if his other features had not compensated so well for it. He was naturally dark-skinned, being of French Mediterranean descent. He had very straight dark-brown hair and high cheek bones that accented that beautiful mouth. His mouth was wide and his lips were thick and long and spoke of an unmitigated sensuality. He stood almost six feet tall and weighed 185.

That night in the bar he wore blue jeans and a white sweat shirt that I still have, though it is riddled with holes and torn and can only barely be called a garment today. Even though I highly suspected that it was useless for me to do so, I went over next to him and stood in the way that hopeful gay men do in hopeless gay bars, and I watched him closely from the corner of my eye to see if there was any hint of an opportunity that I might be able to strike up a conversation with him.

But my instincts, so wrong about everything else, in a case like this were always right on the money. Trying to talk to him was useless. It was like I was in another dimension—as though I weren't there at all—because he didn't notice me. I could have spontaneously combusted; he would not have noticed. Years later, lying in bed late one night, we laughed about that. We would lie in bed at night and hold hands and talk ourselves to sleep. He told me that he never would have noticed me in a million years because I wasn't his type. If he hadn't had AIDS, he said, he never would have noticed I was even alive.

I saw him several times around town over the years. But in all the times I saw him after that first night, I never got his attention not even for a second. I could not get his attention that night. Not until after the epidemic began, and when so many things changed.

I have the memories and the things like his clothes and photographs that stimulate them. But now I look at them and instead think about the hundreds of thousands of people now dead of AIDS. I think about their lovers, their friends, and their families, and the millions of people whose lives have now been touched. And I wonder, *Where does all their pain go?*

## A GLIMPSE OF THE FUTURE

In April 1985 Larry Kramer's *The Normal Heart* opened off-Broadway. It is an incredibly intense play dramatizing the founding of Gay Men's Health Crisis. The lead role, Ned Weeks, was patterned on the play's author and was played by actor Brad Davis. The first night I went to see the play, I was with Rodger McFarlane. After the play we went backstage so that Rodger could speak to some people. I sat down on a bench and watched everyone chat after the performance.

The first time I saw Brad Davis was on a movie screen in the film *Midnight Express* when I was 22 years old. Like so many other gay men, I was attracted to him. The homoerotic scenes from the film, played in a time when such a thing was barely thinkable, caused every gay man with enough money to go to a movie to see it at least twice. His magnitude as an actor was greatly multiplied for gay men, and it is safe to characterize Brad as a gay icon because of *Midnight Express*, which was in 1977. In

1979 I saw Brad again, only this time it was in a very small restaurant in the Village called David's Pot Belly near the Cherry Lane Theater. He sat in a booth next to me, eating his dinner before going on stage in *Entertaining Mr. Sloane*. I was so excited, I could barely eat. I always have a book when I eat alone, but I couldn't concentrate on it even though I wanted him to think that I was. He was so close, I could have easily reached over and touched him just to tell him I admired him. *Excuse me…,* I kept thinking to myself, and then I couldn't think of anything else I would say. I was sure that this happened to him a lot, so I went back to work on my omelet, while out of the corner of my eye, I watched him work on his.

Then backstage at *The Normal Heart* I found myself at the same loss I had been that night in David's Pot Belly. When Rodger, at 6 foot 5, brought over this little guy to meet me (Brad was only about 5 foot 8 on a good day, only his intensity managed to make him taller) and introduced us, Brad shook my hand and gave me a curt nod; I couldn't think of a single thing to say. We did not exchange a single word.

## OPRAH

Six months after I began working at GMHC, in October 1985, I got a call from the producer of *Oprah*. He said that they were doing a show on AIDS discrimination and asked if I would come and be on the panel of guests. The producer's name was Bill Rizzo. I had dated a Billy Rizzo in college, but this didn't sound like him, and I couldn't exactly ask him if we had slept together in college. We made the arrangements for my trip to

Chicago, where I would fly out for the day just for the show, which was filmed live, and then fly back the same day. Other guests were to be Bobby Reynolds, a PWA activist from San Francisco, and a 12-year-old boy from Indiana named Ryan White, who got AIDS through a blood transfusion. As it turned out, Ryan White fell ill and was unable to be there.

When I arrived I discovered that the producer, Bill Rizzo, was after all the same Billy Rizzo I had dated in college. We had both grown up a bit but not so much that we didn't scream when we saw each other. Years later Billy died, and I had heard that Oprah had been close to him, so I sent her a note, but I got back a white card with a handwritten "Nice to hear from you!" which is I guess what most people get, since it didn't seem an appropriate response to a sympathy note.

While I went into the green room, we caught up as best we could with dozens of people standing around. I was introduced to Bobby Reynolds, a hard-boiled activist with a short haircut who I could tell was the kind of radical, flannel-shirted San Francisco activist who would have little use for me. I also met a woman who I can best describe as fawn-like. Her name was Amy Sloan, an Indiana housewife, and she was taking Ryan White's place on the show. Both she and Bobby had AIDS.

Oprah came in and asked if I was nervous. This was a funny question for me. A few months back I would have been scared out of my wits. I had been in my job for only three months when the Rock Hudson announcement made this kind of thing routine. Now I wasn't nervous at all, just anxious to get it over with. Oprah asked if I wanted makeup. I told her that I wanted every bit as much as she had on, and she laughed and took me to the makeup man. He asked me what I wanted, and I told him I would settle for getting rid of the circles under my eyes. He said he'd try, and he made me look passable, though there was no question that Oprah was still wearing more makeup than I was. Afterward I went back to the green room, getting to know my fellow guests. And that was when I got to know one of the most special people I had ever met in my life—Amy Sloan.

In the early 1980s Amy had needed a transfusion during a medical procedure. One of the units of blood she received had been donated by a gay man who had the virus. It was before the HIV antibody test was developed and licensed to screen blood. Years after she recovered from her surgery, Amy found that she was pregnant. A day after the happy news, she got the bad news. The doctors told Amy she had AIDS.

Amy was then faced with a terrible decision, one that was rare in 1985 and that I would never want to make, but today women have to make it all the time. Fortunately, today a woman can elect to take an antiretroviral such as AZT and apparently reduce the chances of her child being born with the virus. Then, there was no AZT. Amy chose to have her baby. He was born HIV-negative. Amy was 24 years old.

She was a wonderful woman and a great mother. She was brave to do what she did. Amy loved her baby enough to take the chance with him despite what it might mean to both of them. She gave him his life. Amy was one of the few people in my life I loved from the moment I met her. She was pretty, with brown eyes and brown hair and beautiful skin. She was tall. She was practical. She had been a dental hygienist who had had to leave her profession upon discovery of her condition.

During the call-in portion of the Oprah show, people questioned whether there ought to be quarantine for PWAs. I started to field the question, but yielded to Amy when I saw her back straighten up at the mere suggestion. I was only a lawyer fighting for my clients' rights; she was a mother fighting for the right to be with her child.

Amy was diagnosed with pneumocystis pneumonia, but the gay man from whom she had gotten HIV was still not sick with a diagnosis of AIDS. That was only one of the many mysteries of this insidious disease. Amy was very collected on *Oprah*. She affirmed that she had the support of family and friends. She deserved it. The most painful part for her, she said, was what was going to happen to her family if she died. Though a physical contrast to Bobby Reynolds, together they spoke the same language. Oprah used the term AIDS victim. She asked, "Do you feel like a victim?"

"I don't like the word *victim,*" said Amy. Bobby nodded. "A lot of times when people talk to me they treat me like an innocent victim. We are all battling the same thing," she said. "We are all innocent."

Call-in talk shows usually do not bring to the fore the nation's most enlightened group of people. *Oprah* was no exception. One caller stated, "I'm just upset about everything that's happened. I'm pretty open-minded, but I think something should be done about the gays. They are not coming up with anything quick enough. They prosecute drunk drivers. They are going to need to prosecute gays for spreading AIDS. I'm afraid to leave my home." This woman represented everything that was typical in the face of the epidemic. She was afraid, and she was reacting to the epidemic out of that fear. She blamed gays, yet Amy, with so much at risk, did not. The scariest thing in this statement, however, was that the woman considered herself "open-minded." Then she asked something that was often asked by frightened people.

"Why don't we have quarantines for this?

"Because we're not gonna do it. I'm not gonna let someone quarantine me," shouted Amy. Amy was a great AIDS activist. She could say everything more clearly and plainly in language everyone could understand.

After the show Amy and her husband and I shared a limo, which dropped me off downtown. I went shopping on Michigan Avenue to kill time before catching my flight home. It was a balmy day in Chicago. Naturally, a wind blew. I went into an exclusive men's shop to buy a tie I couldn't afford, and the salesman asked me if I hadn't been on *Oprah* that morning. "Yep," I said hopefully, "I was." He didn't discount the tie.

I went home to New York. The next day was troublesome at work. I had several unpleasant things to deal with, including a cable show I had gotten scheduled to do for New York state assemblyman Dick Gottfried. The format was to be a show featuring a PWA who had been fired from his job because he had AIDS. Another guest would be his doctor, and there would be call-ins. Again with the call-ins. It was a show I was sure no one would watch, and I was tired and didn't want to do it. To make it less appealing than it already was, complications had arisen with respect to the show.

In the late afternoon I got a call from communications director Lori Behrman. The show might be canceled because the studio where it was to be filmed wouldn't allow a PWA inside. The crew was upset. It looked like a no go. There were a lot of emotional phone calls back and forth. They would have to look for another studio. I secretly hoped that the show would be canceled. After all, I thought, how many people would be seeing a cable show hosted by a New York state assemblyman? I wasn't feeling well. I had come down with a cold. I hadn't been sleeping well, and my pace had been hectic. I had been in umpteen hospitals, my resistance was down, and I was catching everything I could in the way of infections, probably, I guessed, because I had no immune system. I still did not know whether I harbored the virus myself.

I saw no reason to take an HIV test (actually, then it was still called HTLV-III) when it was developed, and in fact it was the conventional wisdom and advice of AIDS service organizations like Gay Men's Health Crisis, AIDS Project Los Angeles, and the San Francisco AIDS Foundation to counsel people away from taking the test. During my appearance on *Oprah,* I sat next to Dr. Harold Jaffe of the Centers for Disease Control and stated that it was my position that people should not take an HTLV-III test. Dr. Jaffe hated this position. But what was the point of a test in 1985? It meant that a person would go through the trauma only to find out that he or she had the virus and would ultimately get a set of opportunistic infections that would kill. There were no such things as antiretrovirals like AZT or ddI, and protease inhibitors were still 11 years away. The only thing gained by taking a test would be knowledge, but in my mind a little knowledge was a dangerous thing, no doubt about it. Epidemiologists would have a better picture of the epidemic. A heavy price for me would come with that knowledge. Some people argued that knowing you were positive meant that you would then have safer sex, knowing you were infected. This seemed just downright silly since in my mind; there wasn't a person in America who shouldn't be having safe sex. Meanwhile, taking a test would mean that the results would be documented in my medical records that I had the virus, and that would make me a target for discrimination. I remember when one day a woman did call me and tell me that she had taken a test because she was concerned about her status. Thankfully, she found that she tested HIV-negative. However, when she went to later apply for an insurance policy, the company looked at her medical records. Recorded there was the fact that she had taken an HIV test. They told her that they would not insure her because she had taken an HIV test and therefore she must be engaged in activities that were high-risk, thereby making her an insurance risk. For me, at that time an HIV test would ruin everything.

Of course, the upside would be that I might find out I did not have the virus. That was the gamble. But even if I were HIV-negative, it was too heavy a price to pay. I'm not sure I wanted to know that I was negative. I'm not sure what that would have meant to me then. Granted, it would be some reassurance. It would also feel like a betrayal to every PWA I had known as a client and to my coworkers and to my friends. That is a perceived burden that would only increase with time. And then too I wasn't so sure about my status. I had never been promiscuous. I had led a dating life but not a life of going out for sex. But I knew a lot of my dead clients had been conservative also. Some of them had been in what they thought were monogamous relationships. Some of them had engaged in unsafe sex only one or two times in their lives. And I knew that I had been unsafe with Todd in the early 1980s. That memory waved like a red flag in front of me every time I thought about taking the test. After all, if I took the test and was positive, it would be me, not some PWA, who this film crew wouldn't want on the set.

I wanted to cancel the whole damned talk show. Every hour the telephone rang with an update. They were trying to persuade the staff. They were trying to find another studio. It was the classic example of a situation where all the discrimination laws in the world aren't going to help you when there is a time frame that doesn't allow a lawsuit. Finally, they told us that they were ready to do the show, which was to be broadcast live from another studio in New York.

The studio was located somewhere near Union Square. Beforehand, because I was tired, I went home and napped, waking up with only enough time to jump into a tie and sports jacket and get to the studio. I had pillow hair so I slicked it back with gel—there was no time for a shower. I washed my face, but it was puffy from sleep and the onset of a cold, and there was a crease on my cheek that was a cast of the wrinkled sheets. I was sure it would be gone by time I got to the studio, but it did flag my confidence just a bit. I arrived at the studio and waited in a dark hallway for the show to begin. They said that they were ready, and I walked onto the set to find the doctor, a woman physician well-known in Manhattan for treating PWAs, and the PWA himself, Joseph. He was the man I had been so smitten with in Uncle Charlie's bar all those years ago. Here was the most beautiful man I had ever seen. He was the talk-show focus.

He was the man brought in to talk about being fired from his job because of AIDS discrimination and, ironically, had been victimized by AIDS discrimination that very afternoon. He was nervous. When the show ran our names under our talking heads, his said just "Joseph." He declined to use his last name.

I was a bit shaken by the sight of him. I hadn't known he had AIDS. He didn't look like he had AIDS. He looked just the way he looked back in Uncle Charlie's, except that the six or seven years had given him a more mature beauty. By no means had AIDS diminished the grandeur of that smile or that face or the magnitude of his appeal. He was still the most striking man I had ever seen in my entire life.

We met there on that talk show, and throughout the entire show I was absolutely mesmerized by his presence, which the camera recorded faithfully. I had trouble concentrating on the fact that we were on cable television and with other people— that we had a purpose that was something other than my actually getting to talk to him. I wanted to take him by the hand and lead him off the set and talk to him and tell him about the fact that I had admired and remembered him for years. As he spoke he would sometimes toss his head back and smile, and I would feel myself drawn in to his beauty. My infatuation with him is apparent now in watching a tape of the show. I gaped at him with a kind of stupid expression, the hangover of my nap still having its effect on me, now combined with dumbstruck lovesickness. Even with other people talking to me and directing questions to me, I answered looking only at him. I was grateful when during the call-in portion of the show he would get to answer the caller's question, because it gave me an excuse for staring at him.

The show began by noting the fact that the studio where the show was to originally be filmed would not allow Joseph in. Clearly, he was disturbed and angry. The experience of being turned away because of who and what he was had been devastating and humiliating. He had after all already lost his job because of discrimination when it was discovered he had AIDS. He was the man who had called me six months before for help, and I had turned him down, and he had hung up on me. All the pieces came together for me as he told his story of discrimination. Oh. Oops. Big oops. The show lasted one hour, and afterward we said good night to Assemblyman Gottfried and to the doctor. We walked outside together to catch cabs. I tried desperately to engage him in some small talk without any real thought as to what I would do if he responded with any interest in me. I had no plan if he had responded by asking me if I wanted to go for coffee. But I needn't have worried. He was almost as oblivious to me and my presence as he had been in Uncle Charlie's so many years before. He commented on how hurtful the reaction of the studio was. I asked if he wanted to go get a cup of coffee or something somewhere. No, he said, he just wanted to go home. He raised his hand and a Marathon cab immediately stopped at the curb, and he said good night. I stood there on 14th Street feeling like Nerd Lawyer from Hell. I raised my hand for a cab; of course, one didn't materialize. I just stood there like some gay urban statue of liberty. I should just give up on trying to attract men, I thought. I went home and nursed my cold, struck by the loss of this man, not only to me but to himself.

Many months later after we were living together, we looked back on this and laughed. One day his old roommate, Bobby, called the apartment, and I answered the telephone. They hadn't spoken in many months, and Bobby naturally asked who had answered the phone. Joe told him my name and told him we were living together now. "Isn't that the guy who wouldn't help you?" asked Bobby. "What happened?"

"I fell in love with him," said Joe, smiling.

But after the show that night I did not see him again until a few weeks later when he began volunteering at the agency. GMHC, like many other AIDS organizations, has an annual AIDS walk to raise money for the organization. The walk was run by a team of consultants put together by Craig Miller and Richard Zeichik, two men who have probably together raised more money for AIDS than anyone else in New York, Atlanta, San Francisco, or Los Angeles. Joe, having lost his job as a result of being fired, was working for them. I began to see him at staff meetings, which we regularly held at GMHC. These meetings, which I usually dreaded, I began to look forward to, just so that I could see him sitting down an aisle of seats or at the end of a row. He usually sat in back, which was really annoying because I always had to make an excuse to turn around, and in the course of a one-hour meeting there are only so many excuses for turning completely around to stare at someone in back of you. Then one day I noticed a small star-like bruise on his forehead. I buried my suspicion, but after a few weeks asked someone at the agency who knew him whether his was KS. My heart broke a little when I was told that Joe did have KS, and there it was on his face. The memory of Richard presented itself again like Banquo's ghost every time I ever looked at his lesion again. At least I had finally met him. Now if only I could get his attention.

# CHAPTER 7 : 1986

*18,814 new cases of AIDS were diagnosed*
*11,875 more people died*
*A cumulative total of 41,088 cases were diagnosed*
*24,208 people were dead of AIDS in America*

A few months later in early spring I found myself having a bad day at the office. The first year of doing this full time was taking its toll, and I learned that it pays to take a break in the middle of the day when I need it. I decided to take a walk around the neighborhood just to get a breather. Turning a corner, I quite literally ran into Joe. I blurted out a hello. He stopped to talk to me, saying that he was out for a walk because he didn't feel he could any longer handle the work with the consultants. We chatted about our mutual frustrations with work, and then I did something that required the summons of all my courage. It was not something I had done successfully with very many men on very many occasions. I asked him out. I suggested that we have dinner together soon. We made plans for the following week.

I walked back to my office, elated on the one hand and profoundly disturbed by what I had done. I told myself that despite
my strong attraction to this man, I wanted only to be friends and
that this wasn't really a date. Who in the world, I asked myself,
would date someone with AIDS? It wasn't as if we could ever
consummate a relationship like this. It would be seen as the ul-
timate in self-destruction. So it wasn't a date; I just wanted to be
this man's friend.

The night of our dinner, April 12, 1986, I spent hours getting
ready, changing clothes several times, wanting to look good because, I told myself, I always wanted to look good. We went to
an Italian restaurant on the upper west side near my apartment.
I was a nervous wreck and don't have any recollection of what
we had talked about except that I had a beard then and he told
me that he didn't like beards. I didn't smoke, but he had ciga-
rettes, so I started smoking them. There didn't exactly seem to
be any real chemistry at work. Maybe he was just too handsome
for me to get to the point sensibly where chemistry had a
chance. Or maybe the fact that he had AIDS kind of quelled any
chemistry brewing. But it wasn't a disaster date either, and we
both made it through to the end to say good night, and once
again I watched him get into a cab and speed away from me. The
next morning I shaved off my beard.

Over the next several days I did not hear from him again, and
I felt that I had expended all my bravado in asking him out in
the first place. When two weeks later he called and left a message on my machine, I assumed it was a man named Joseph from
my church and didn't hurry to call back.

Joe had begun volunteering for the GMHC hotline. I had to

pass the hotline office to get to my own, and I would make excuses to walk by there as many times as possible in an afternoon
on the days he volunteered. We'd wave if he was on the phone,
which was almost always the case. One day he stopped me to ask
why I had never returned his call. Slack-mouthed, I mumbled an
excuse at first not understanding what he had meant. Then I realized that it was the wrong Joseph I was thinking about when
I failed to return the call. It wasn't the Joseph from my church;
it was this Joseph.

Another hotline activity involved handing out literature on
street corners, and it was staffed by volunteers from the hotline.
The following Saturday, I was on my way to do a will consultation. I liked walking from the west side to the east side through
Central Park and set out along 72nd Street. At Columbus Avenue Joe was standing at a hotline table with his jacket in hand,
getting ready to go home to his east-side apartment. When I said
hello, he turned around and kissed me hello on my mouth. It
was the briefest flutter of a kiss—like a butterfly crossing my lips.
I was rattled by it. I had never kissed anyone with AIDS before.
I didn't want to think about what that meant.

We decided to walk across the park together. He was going to
East 64th Street and I was going to East 58th Street. I can remember that it was a windy spring day with just a hint of May,
my favorite month in New York. It was the most self-conscious
walk I had ever taken. I felt clumsy and awkward, searching for
something to talk about. I tried again to explain why I hadn't
called him back. Later in another one of those hand-holding
nights before sleep, I confessed to him that during that walk I
believed I was the quintessential oaf, worried that he must have

thought me terribly unsophisticated, not on the level of other men he had gone out with from the Studio 54 set. He confided to me that he was fearful I was thinking of him that he was just another dumb, uneducated actor-model-waiter, making *him* feel terribly self-conscious during the entire walk. For a simple walk in the park we generated a lot of angst.

When we got to the east side of the park, we arranged another dinner date. I was sorry to see this walk end because I really wanted to spend more time with him, but I was also anxious for the end because, as I had hoped during the entire walk, the butterfly kiss made another guest appearance on my lips, this time less tentative.

A few days later we went. We went to more dinners several times over the next several days. After one of the dinners he came back to my apartment to say good night. I asked him if I could kiss him good night. That was the first time we kissed more than hello and good-bye. We kissed hard and long, and I couldn't breathe. The promise of those sensual lips lived up to itself and more. I could have stood there all night and done nothing else. We paused and held each other for a moment, both of our bodies rigid against one another. "That wasn't so bad," I said.

"No," he replied and swallowed hard, "it wasn't so bad." Slowly we let each other go. I think we each wanted to be with one another, but we wanted to be with our own thoughts more. We said good night.

I now went to therapy regularly, helping me in answering some of the many questions that came to my mind in working in AIDS. Needless to say, my therapist, Jim, was fascinated by the turn of events involving Joe. We talked about only this, trying to feel out my motivation. We both wanted to be sure I wasn't bent on self-destruction. I explained to Jim that I was falling in love with this man. It was not a desire to die; I didn't want to die. I had seen so much of the death and destruction of AIDS that dying that way was my second worst nightmare. But my first nightmare was to have my life and my destiny and my happiness controlled by something so small as an insidious virus. I didn't want that virus telling me who I could and could not fall in love with; it would be ceding too much control to the enemy. I explained that if I let that happen, then I would be a victim of AIDS, not because I contracted the disease but because I stood by helplessly while it ravaged my life. I would be damned if I would let the virus rob me of my happiness.

Jim was worried. I had told him that Joe had a bad KS lesion on the roof of his mouth. "Aren't you afraid of that?" he asked. He wondered if it might not shed blood cells that would make Joe's saliva infectious and possibly could cause me to become infected. I said I just didn't know. Finally, Jim, like a priest in a confessional, bestowed a blessing by conferring his opinion that I was not being self-destructive but that I needed to be careful nonetheless. Careful? Careful? Now what in the world could careful mean in this situation? I didn't know. Sure there was "safe sex," which broke down sex into categories of low risk, moderate risk, and lots of risk. So what does that mean really? When you are in bed with someone and you have to consider risk categories in the grips of passion, it sort of takes the passion out of the equation. Moreover, I knew that safe sex didn't mean absolutely safe sex. There was no zero-sum risk to anything.

Joe and I were invited to a Martha Graham Company dance performance by Allen Wallace, the man who had been Richard's care partner. He had become boyfriends with my best friend, Michael, and we were joining them at the theater. Joe and I were meeting there as well. I waited outside and saw him walking up the street with an air of casual elegance that he had mastered so well. He wore a white shirt, white linen slacks, and a thin, blue, unconstructed jacket. It looked as if those clothes had been made only for him. After the performance we went to a brief dinner and then back to my apartment. Sitting on the couch, we talked until late into the night. And then he kissed me again.

After some time we sat with our arms around one another, not saying anything, our clothes somewhat a mess. I reached over and whispered in his ear to ask him if he would like to stay over. He held me close and was quiet for a moment. Then he whispered in my ear and told me that he had never been with a "well person" since he had been diagnosed. Whispering like this seemed to be the only way we could have this conversation. I thought about what he had said for a moment. I told him that I had never been with a "sick person" either, getting a little hung up on those words. We paused, and then he began to remove my clothing and removed his. He turned and walked up the stairway to my bed. I can remember the sight of his silky smooth back as he went up the stairs and my feeling of relief and the burial of my fear—and we went to bed. It was a pretty wonderful night, and in the dark I couldn't see any small lesion, nor could I see the threats involved in sleeping with someone with AIDS. For a night we could just forget about everything else and hide it all in the dark while we explored each other's bodies and passion. There wasn't even enough light or space for any fear to creep in and disturb us.

In the morning my eyes opened with a start because I knew that my arm was around someone. I didn't move. I stared out into space and asked myself what had I done. Up until now I had worried about everyone I had ever been with—did they have AIDS and could I have gotten it? Now, here I was, knowingly in bed with someone who had AIDS. Falling in love with someone who was going to die. I will never know the reason, but the fear I had experienced about past boyfriends never came back to me again. I wasn't afraid about getting AIDS from him; we were safe. I was afraid I would lose him. I turned and looked at him, and he opened his eyes. I don't know if I saw fear in his eyes or my own fear reflected. I don't know if he ever sensed the panic I felt. I never asked him during one of those late night talks we would have later.

This began the most wonderful and awful time of my life. It was like the last meal granted one on death row. It was everything I wanted, only to be taken away from me by the inevitable fate of what was bound to occur. I was never in denial about what was to come. I did have a sense of angry defiance about it, though. I felt like we were getting cheated.

We had decided that for as long as possible we should try and keep our liaison a secret. In 1986 a PWA with a well person was virtually unheard-of, and people would feel threatened by it. Even if not threatening, it would compel people to talk about our personal lives, a situation with which neither of us was particularly comfortable.

GMHC was a small operation in those days. We were still housed on West 18th Street in Chelsea in a small two-story office of a few thousand square feet. The office occupied the second and third floors over a restaurant. There was a small kitchen off the reception area on the second floor where everyone went for coffee or to microwave their lunch. Typically, it was the hub of activity in the small agency, with staff and clients and volunteers to congregate by the proverbial water cooler. Several weeks into my relationship with Joseph, I was pouring a cup of coffee in the kitchen when the voice of Barry Davidson boomed from a corner of the crowded room. The noise in that room was typically on the level of any New York subway. There was a constant dither of multiple conversations simultaneously occurring on any number of subjects, like priests chanting separate prayers. In the story of my life, I had always promised, Barry Davidson would be played by Bea Arthur. Needless to say, when Barry spoke his words, the room came to a complete stop.

"I heard dish about you on Fire Island this weekend," he said with pursed lips and a very knowing glance at me. His eyes were lit by the fire of really good gossip. They were like two glowing flares.

I sensibly stopped pouring coffee so that I did not spill it all over my hand. I suspected that somehow someone knew the truth about me and Joe.

"Well, Barry," I said to a now-captivated room, "it could hardly be accurate dish. I have been to Fire Island only once in my life, and that was in 1977. I didn't even like it then. I haven't been back since. Any dish you heard could only be unfounded rumor." I thought I had smartly dealt with that.

But Barry was not daunted. "Well, I did hear about you and your new boyfriend," he said.

I froze. I didn't have much of a comeback to that. I believe I then just froze in one of those Nancy Reagan type of smiles and said something clever and witty like, "Boyfriend?"

"Yes," he said, "and I want you to know that I think it is just wonderful."

Then I knew that Barry did indeed know. I bowed my head to my coffee and left the room to my office. My assistant, a 45-year-old man (who will be played by Eve Arden), looked at me as I rushed by and slammed my door to get on the phone to call Joseph, who was not home. But before I got out of that kitchen, I could feel everyone beginning to form their questions to Barry about the who and the what.

Later that day Joe came into my office, and I told him what had happened. John sat in an office situated before mine so that to enter mine you had to walk through his. John had seen Joe come in. I told him very softly about Barry and the kitchen. He didn't really have time to talk—he was late for the hotline—but whispered "It's OK" in my ear and then gave me a long and caring kiss good-bye.

"Bye," he said loudly.

"Bye then," I said. After he left, John Mokricky poked his head through my door. "My," he said, "that sounded like a nice good-bye kiss."

Word was out. When people can hear a kiss, it is hard to keep a secret. But not everyone felt the way Barry felt. In fact, hardly anyone. It was truly ironic that in an AIDS organization in 1986, there would be so little empathy for a sero-discordant couple, which today is not uncommon at all. People asked me if I was trying to kill myself. People were upset. People were not particularly nice and were not at all sensitive in expressing their opinions. He's going to die, people would say, as if that were the sole criteria for deciding whether you could fall in love with someone. Do you want to be infected? Are you crazy? I could not have much response. No I didn't want to get infected, and no I didn't want him to die. Nor if I had my wishes, would he. No, I didn't think I was crazy. It seemed pointless to try to explain.

But I knew something very definite. I wanted to make my choices in my life; I didn't want HIV to make them for me. If I ignored my feelings for Joe, tossed aside the history of interest in him that I had, forgot how much I liked being with him solely because he had AIDS, then I would be letting the virus take control of my life in a way that was unacceptable to me. I had never fallen in love before. I was not going to give the virus the satisfaction of taking this away from me. I did not choose these circumstances; they chose me.

It was not like a Hollywood script where people respond by saying something like, "Oh, of course, you are right." Or "It is your life, you can lead it any way you want." Or "Gee, what you say is thoughtful and deeper than I have considered this before." They just looked at me like I was crazy. I don't think people wanted to accept this because it meant accepting a future for HIV in their lives and their decisions as well. While at the time there were not many sero-discordant couples, it was perfectly obvious that if the epidemic continued to grow the way it was, there would be a time when we would all be faced with decisions like these. And since I did not know at the time whether I had the virus, then, I reasoned, Joe's having AIDS would mean little if I had already been infected. None of us knew. I knew only that I was doing what I needed to do to survive, as ironic as that may sound. If I caved in to the virus on this point, I would never be able to continue my work. And more important to me, I would never be able to think of myself as anything other than a coward. I may not have much of the countenance of a brave man, but one thing I can say about myself in looking back to those days: I am no coward. Prior to the epidemic, I always believed that I was.

We began to date regularly and went through the fun and trials that newly dating couples have. I began to forget that he was sick and I was well. With the exception of some days where he didn't feel so well and the small Kaposi's sarcoma lesion on his forehead, it began to feel like a normal relationship. Reality would come crashing through when one night while kissing his ear, I discovered a new lesion on the backside of it. Another appeared on his inner thigh. But those intrusions didn't stop us from getting more involved in the daily routine of our living. I don't remember when I told him I loved him, but we told each other often once we took the plunge.

## LOCKUP

Riker's Island is a prison facility in New York. To get there you have to catch a bus from the east side by the 59th Street bridge, and after what seems like a long time you end up in what is unmistakably a prison.

During the summer there had been some activity in the prison, noted in the press, in the AIDS ward. The guys locked up there wanted better treatment and wanted to see a lawyer. I didn't take much note of this until I got a request in my office from someone in the AIDS ward to please come out there. In the spring of 1986 *The New York Times* carried a story about the work of the volunteer lawyers and my office at GMHC. It was on the front page of the Metropolitan section of the paper and carried a not-so-flattering photograph of me. Apparently, someone on the island had seen it.

I had to make an application to the prison system for a pass, which bureaucracy being what it is, took quite a while. I wanted to look very unlawyer-like for my photograph that would be affixed to the identification card I would need, so I wore my favorite Hawaiian shirt. Once I got my pass it looked like one for an island tour, which in a way it was. I scheduled my first visit and made the trek to the island.

I had been in a prison only once before—in high school on a field trip with a civics class. I didn't remember much about it except that there was one prisoner who was extremely indignant, and in a question-answer session appeared to be fairly unstable. But I did not recall the minute aspects of prison life I picked up on Riker's Island. Entry into the prison naturally begins with going through several locked doors. Going through a couple of these is no big deal, but by the time you have entered a dozen or so doors, for which there are elaborate procedures for unlocking and locking them, a sense of claustrophobia begins to overtake one. The guards are not greeters; they are guards. I felt as if the word FAG was imprinted on my forehead by the way each one of them regarded me. I said "Hi" to everyone, as if it were my first day at camp. This was universally greeted by a stony silence, no one responding "Hi" back. I began to temper my outgoing nature, reserving myself to nods to each guard. They didn't change their stance; they merely glared at that word on my forehead. As I passed each door I began to have the feeling that if they could, they would just leave me in there and not let me out. I began to feel very, very vulnerable and very, very tiny. I had never seen so many guns in my life.

Going through several locked doors, I made my way to the prison hospital. Once there I got into an elevator to take it up to the AIDS ward. I have never liked elevators in the first place, much less one with locks on it. Once at the top I made it through yet another pair of guarded, locked doors and finally presented myself at the door of the AIDS ward. The guard looked up at me. "Hi." No one accompanied me inside.

The first thing one can say about it was that it was dirty. There was little to indicate that this was a ward in a hospital. It was nothing more than a collection of cells. "AIDS ward" was misleading. It was more like an AIDS warehouse. Some of the men were very, very sick; others were not, but were HIV-positive. They were an even mix of Hispanics, blacks, and Caucasians, and there were very rough, butch guys, and others who were polishing their nails and carrying on in the campiest ways. Everyone just kind of stopped what they were doing and looked at me. I looked for a place to set my things down, but there wasn't much space for anything. There was a bad feeling in my stomach. I didn't know how to begin; this wasn't exactly covered in any of my law school courses.

The second thing I can say about it is that it was very, very frightening to be locked up in this cell block and be the only person who didn't have AIDS. I don't mean that it was frightening in the sense that I was afraid of contagion; I knew better than that. But there was something very eerie about being confined with a lot of people who you know are going to die. And they know that they are probably going to die in there. They know that you are not. They are the desperate of the desperate. And it was very sad to see all these wrecked lives, all in this spot, with not much in common except that they had committed a crime and they were all going to suffer an unpleasant death in what was unquestionably a death row.

I looked at each of the guys, and they looked back at me. "Hi," I said. As I gazed at each one I couldn't help wondering what their crime had been. Having never met one, I wondered if anyone was a murderer. I didn't particularly want to meet one now. Clearly, they all had a capacity for some kind of violence, though by looking at some of them, this was hard to believe. With others the look of menace on their faces would have kept me on the other side of the street had I seen them outside of these walls.

One guy came up to me. "Hi," he said. Finally. We introduced ourselves. His name was Angel. He was very personable, and it was hard for me to imagine that he had committed a crime that landed him in here. Fortunately, Angel sort of took charge of things. He said that most of the guys wanted to see me. There were about 20 of them, and 14 of them wanted to talk. It felt like it was going to be a long day. I explained that I was there to write wills for anyone who wanted one done but that I also had an appointment with the deputy warden afterward. I said I would convey any concerns they had about their treatment as people with AIDS.

Angel arranged everyone's appointment and sat down with me first because he wanted to write a will, but he also wanted me to know about some other things—about the trial system and criminal law. I had no way of knowing if everything he told me was true or not. He said that a few months back one of the guys in the ward had a bad case of cryptosporidium, causing severe diarrhea, and that he ended up just shitting all over himself in his bed. Angel said that no one came to change him, and the man became terribly despondent. Since this was not an uncommon story even in the city's hospitals, I wasn't surprised to hear it. But then Angel told me that the man had eventually set himself on fire.

"How long have you been in here?" I asked Angel.

"Ten months," he said.

"Ten months?" I asked. This seemed like a long time to me because I was under the impression that Riker's was a place where people were held until they were through with their trial or to serve short time, but anything that was a major sentence meant being sent to a penitentiary. "Isn't your lawyer doing anything?"

I asked this question not really wanting to know the answer because I didn't know anything about criminal law to speak of and didn't want to know anything about it. I made it clear to the guys when I sat down that I was not a criminal lawyer and that I would not be seeking to represent them in any way with regard to their charges but would only be addressing issues that related to AIDS.

"Lawyers don't come in here," said Angel.

"What about Legal Aid?" I asked. "What about the public defender's office?"

"Nope," said Angel. "They're all afraid to come in here. Even the guards are afraid to come in here." Then Angel told me something that made me angry.

"Some of these guys…see that guy over there. He has been in here for 19 months on an arraignment. He hasn't even had his day in court."

"Nineteen months on an arraignment?"

"Yeah," said Angel, "and that guy over there has been in 15 months. See, they come and get them for their court date, and they take them into the van and drive them to court. Then here at the island, it gets recorded that they went to court. But when they get there, they either get put into the pen, where they wait all day without getting into court, or sometimes they're just left in the hot van because no one will touch them to bring them in."

"It's a hell of a thing," said Angel, "to have a fever and be cuffed in the back of a hot van all day." Angel, who had been somewhat lighthearted in everything he had told me, was so serious now and spoke with so much conviction that I felt certain he was telling the truth, at least about sitting in the van. "The guards at the court won't touch these guys, so they sit there, but they don't get to go into court. Then they come back here."

"And their lawyers don't come in here?" I asked, incredulous.

"No, that's why we wanted you to come when we read about you in the paper," Angel took the back of his hand and tapped my shoulder, a gesture meant to say "Get it?"

Then he told me about the refrigerator that was taken away from them. Some of the guys, he said, needed to drink Ensure, but they didn't have a refrigerator to keep it cold. There had been one, but it was taken away. They also wanted a microwave.

The list of wants grew, and several of the guys talked to me at once.

Dazed, I did a few will interviews with some of the guys. During Angel's, I got the courage up to tactfully ask why he was in the slammer. "Burglary," he told me. I was kind of relieved to hear that, since it didn't feel like a violent crime to me, and I had developed a fondness for Angel. I finished the will interviews, some of which were about assets in their estates that had some fascinating histories, and explained that I would need to come back with the prepared instruments for them to sign and that I would return as soon as I could. They assured me they would be there. Clearly, there was no reason to believe otherwise.

I went to the door and gave the signal to the guard that I wanted to leave. It was with a great sense of relief when he came to let me out. On some level I had a deep-seated paranoia that he wouldn't respond. On my way to the elevator I had to pass by the ward's medical staff, a doctor. He looked sad and gray and tired and disinterested. We didn't speak. Now I felt as if the guards and the staff were Them and I had, by consorting with the inmates, become part of Us. If the doctor hadn't had on the white coat and stethoscope, it would not have occurred to me that he was a physician. He was smoking a cigarette, one of those incongruities that always unnerves me: a doctor who smokes. It's like watching an obese person eat mayonnaise. But even more unnerving was the fact that he was doing it inside the hospital ward. As the door shut behind me and the elevator doors opened, I sensed a little of the gloom I felt leave me. With each succeeding doorway I went through,

I felt shackles drop from me. I went to my appointment at the deputy warden's office.

The person sitting behind the desk surprised me. She was very pretty with long black hair pinned up in a neat and very restrained French roll. She had perfect dark skin and beautiful eyes. She was African-American. She maintained one expression during our entire interview process—polite indifference.

"Hi," I ventured.

"Hello," she said. She was the hello kind of person.

I thanked her for her time. We discussed the conditions of the AIDS ward. I brought up the refrigerator and the microwave. She said she would see what she could do. I explained the medical reasons that PWAs would need these and other small necessities, which could be easily provided.

Then I brought up the issue of condoms. I cited to her the statistics of the estimated rates of infection for people in New York City and that undoubtedly there were many prisoners in her resident population who were HIV infected and asymptomatic. I explained that condoms could be made available very cheaply.

"We do not condone sexual behavior in the prison. Sexual behavior in prison is not permitted," she said, still with that slight smile on her face. She was very composed.

"Yes," I said. "But still, don't you think that it happens anyway?"

She repeated her previous statement word for word, never changing her tone or her expression.

"Well," I said, "but you know and I know that even though it is not sanctioned, they are doing it like bunnies out there."

She repeated her statement verbatim a third time. I had hit a prison wall.

When I got back to Manhattan and got off the bus, I couldn't shake the feeling of oppression I had left over from the prison. The hateful stares from the guards, the locks, the doors, the genuine fear I had felt, the stupidity of the beautiful deputy warden's statement—all weighed down on me. The bus left me off under the 59th Street bridge, and I walked to Joe's apartment on East 64th Street. I was so happy to find him home. We lay down on his bed, and I told him what it was like. Outside, there was a thunderstorm, and it began to rain. Inside, while I told him about each of the guys and what prison was like, I began to cry.

"Why are you crying?" he asked. I could tell he was annoyed.

"I don't know; it was all just so pathetic. I have never been in a place filled with so much hate and so much hopelessness. I didn't know people could exist that way." I think I was crying because I didn't want to know people could exist that way. I was crying because that day I lost a big chunk of my innocence, and I knew I would never get it back. That's the thing about AIDS: It takes so much away that can never be given back.

"Well," he said, "if you're going to get this upset, I don't want you going back anymore."

"I won't be upset every time," I said defensively. But while I didn't cry every time I went back, I was upset each time I walked in there. Joe held me close and then performed some magic to make me forget about the prison, while outside the spring rain and thunder did their best to keep up. He did it for me, I could tell. He had a fever and didn't feel well. But he knew that he could still make me feel better.

It was several weeks before I was able to schedule another visit to the ward. When I got up there, I was pleased to see that there was a refrigerator and a microwave. It was a little bit cleaner as well, though Angel told me that the cleaning had occurred only for my benefit. Angel signed his will. It was a somber moment for him. The population of the ward had changed somewhat, but those who had met me before were happy to see me again.

The next time I went it was an autumn day; the population had turned over dramatically, and there was a sea change in the mood of the place. I was told that the heat was only turned on for the benefit of my visit. Still, in some areas it felt cold to me. A cockroach crawled onto my jacket. Some of the guys wouldn't come and talk to me at all because there was one prisoner who said they shouldn't talk to the "fag," and so some of the guys stayed away under threat of punishment from the rough guy. Only the original inmates from my first visit came to talk. I left that time, and I never went back.

Many years later when I lived in California, I was driving home from work and heard a report on the news about Riker's Island and the AIDS prison ward. It had expanded dramatically and now included many more people. Members of the prison population, like so many others in the United States, were dying in large numbers of AIDS, and in fact it had become the number one killer of prisoners in New York. And, the report said, condoms were finally being made available.

I smiled, thinking of Angel and how far away those days on Riker's Island seemed to be to me. And then I thought of all the lives lost because of the prison policy. I thought of the deputy warden with her stoic beauty and immovable policy. Once more her words "We do not condone sexual behavior in the prison" went through my head. I wondered how her soul could bear the burden of her inaction—a sin of letting so many men get infected. Once again and for the last time the AIDS prison ward on Riker's Island brought a tear to me eye while I sat there on the Hollywood freeway—3,000 miles away, stuck in traffic with the top down while the sun beat down on my head and I pondered the ignorance that inevitably brought misery to many more lives.

## SURVIVING AND THRIVING

During the summer of 1986 there was a national conference of people with AIDS to be held in San Francisco, and Joe wanted to go alone. But I wheedled until I got my way, and we went together. Earlier in the spring he had gone to Key West with a friend of his from Los Angeles because he wanted to be on his own for a bit and, not wanting to cramp him, I had said I was OK with it, even though I really wanted to go. He ended up calling two days into the trip to ask me to go down and join him, which at that point I couldn't do. So for the trip to San Francisco, I only had to apply a minimal amount of nagging to get my way. We stayed at the St. Francis. We checked in late the day before the conference started and ordered breakfast in bed, which was thrilling. But the trip there seemed to wear Joe down quite a bit, and his mood didn't match my somewhat boisterous spirits.

These AIDS conferences can be bittersweet. I was excited to see that my Oprah buddy, Amy Sloan, was there so I could introduce her to Joe. Bobby Reynolds was also there as well as a host of friends I had come to know in New York, Joe's AIDS gang. Michael Calvert, an old client of mine and a good friend of Joe's, singer and activist Michael Callen, Michael Hirsch, and my friend Jane Rosette. We had met at the People With AIDS Coalition office in New York, where she volunteered as a photographer.

PWAC was an organization formed in New York by a handful of PWAs who wanted to assert their rejection of the assumption that AIDS was an automatic death sentence. They produced a monthly newsletter with treatment tips, home remedies, stories, and, of course, obituaries. Joe was a founding member of the board of directors, and these people had become just about his only friends. He and his friends who were not sick seemed to avoid one another.

PWAC did offer something special—a fraternity based on fatality. Eventually they produced a booklet called *Surviving and Thriving With AIDS,* something which at that time was expressed more as a hope than a reality. On the cover is a photograph of Joe and all the AIDS gang: Michael Calvert, Griffin Gold, Michael Hirsch, and Michael Callen. Today, none of them have survived. Most of them did, however, have their moments when they thrived.

It is a fascinating thing to watch someone struggle for his life. If you aren't involved in the same struggle, then you are truly only someone on the outside, looking in. Though of course in the back of our minds, those of us "at risk" for AIDS had to wonder who was next. Were these PWAs just paving the way for me for the day I would discover my purple lesion or be short of breath and headed for the hospital? They were very brave, these early PWAs, and they were vigilant. It was frustrating to watch them in that strug-

gle and to be able to do so little to help, trying to believe in a notion that they were surviving and thriving with this insidious disease. Jane and I were codependents, helping them try to believe
this, accepting our role as outsiders who couldn't possibly know
what it was like to have AIDS, while at the same time knowing all
too well. The conference presented us with the unfathomable situation of watching a whole roomful of people struggle with their
mortality, watching a disaster unfold and engulf people in slow
motion. Of all the people who created PWAC in New York, and
the greater number of them who were at the national PWAC
conference, none are alive today. Except for myself and Jane.
Hence, the bittersweet nature of the conference.

I was a little anxious in San Francisco because it was the first
trip Joe and I had taken together. The week before we had spent
a wonderful weekend in Amagansett at a friend's house, but this
was the longest period of time we would be spending together.
Joe was very distracted by the conference and by the concentra-
tion on the AIDS part of his life. On the other hand, I was really wanting to be the center of his attention on what I viewed as
a vacation. But the conference focus on mortality and the falla-
cy of surviving and thriving seemed to weigh him down, and he
became moody and sluggish.

While I was in San Francisco I got to visit my friend Neil. It
was odd to spend time with him. We had spent so much time
together as children, but when we graduated from our separate
colleges, he moved to San Francisco and I went to New York.
We didn't have much in common anymore, but we had a loyalty to one another that was based on years of foundation. But
now he represented something to me that I didn't want to deal

with. He had taken the test and discovered he was positive. Now, when I visited with him, all I could think about was that he was going to get sick and die and how I couldn't imagine knowing what that was like. He would tell me I should get tested. I asked him what was the point? It was an unpleasant disagreement. After all, saying that I didn't want to get tested meant that what I was really saying was "I don't want to be like you." And that was the crux of it in a way. I couldn't help feeling as if I was not part of some special fraternal order when I was at the PWAC conference. Jane Rosette and I were the only non-PWAs. Jane is Jewish, and I'm Catholic, so we had a good deal of shared guilt at not being a PWA—we couldn't know how it was for them. But the truth was, I didn't want to know, and Joe and I weren't having the best of times in San Francisco. We didn't spend a great deal of time together on this part of the trip.

When the conference was done Joe and I left San Francisco and drove north through the wine country, staying on the coast for a few extra days. We enjoyed our side trip, and Joe relaxed a little. One evening we ate at a restaurant on the coast that overlooked a dramatic seascape, and it was very romantic. It was our most pleasant evening since being at Amagansett. But the next day he seemed to have trouble breathing and was overwhelmingly tired, and he became sullen.

We flew back to New York, and I was somewhat relieved to send him home and be out from under the strain of not saying the wrong thing at the wrong time and at the same time looking out for him. But the day after we got home he went to the doctor and was admitted to the hospital. It was suspected that he might have pneumocystis pneumonia.

The test for pneumocystis is called a bronchoscopy. It involves shoving a lot of things down one's throat into the breathing passages, where tissue is removed for examination for infection. It is not a fun procedure. Most hospitals in epicenters have become quite proficient at administering them because of sheer volume. Back then, it was hit or miss as to whether you got someone who knew how to do it without causing a great deal of discomfort to the patient. Joe didn't feel he'd been too lucky with this bronchoscopy. It came back positive. He had acquired the opportunistic infection that killed more PWAs than any other.

At that time the treatment protocol for this opportunistic infection was a three-week course of a strong antibiotic. Toward the end of the treatment, during the third week, it is difficult for the patient to eat, having a metallic taste in his mouth, and what goes down usually comes back up. Joe was seeing a doctor who had admitting privileges at Cabrini Hospital, a Catholic institution. I advised the nursing station that I would be spending the night with Joe. While it is a commonplace practice today, at that time it was not. I parenthetically let it be known that if I didn't get my way on this, I was going to throw the biggest diva attack they ever saw, one that would only begin by my hauling in GMHC. The first night I slept sitting up in a chair. The next night, they sent a cot up to Joe's room for me. He experienced a bad time during the third week of medication. I helped him eat that last week. I went to the hospital every day. I helped him bathe. I came in from work one day to find that he had a picture of me stuck to the side of his bed. It made me realize how important it was that we stay together while he was in the hospital. Clearly he thought he might die, but I knew this wasn't the time and I wasn't afraid. One day he lay in bed while I was reading to him. He appeared distracted by something, staring at the ceiling. I stopped reading and looked up, but saw nothing.

"What is it?"

He hesitated before answering. "I see 'The Light,' " he said, referring to the bright, white light so many people who have had near-death experiences have reported. I stared at his face while he continued to stare at the ceiling. Slyly, he shifted his gaze to me and smiled. I didn't think it was funny. Then he got serious and asked me if he had The Look yet. I assured him that he was far way away from The Look and stroked his hair, telling him how handsome he still was. But the conversation was sobering for us both, reminding us that both things would happen. He would see The Light, and even though I wouldn't acknowledge it, eventually he had The Look. But not yet. Upon his discharge from the hospital, he moved in with me.

Life returned to a state of normalcy, though the bout of pneumonia grounded us both to the fact that he was fighting for his life. One night during his hospital stay he insisted that he be allowed to go to the birthday party of his friend David Summers, the fellow who went onto the talk show with me and was threatened with a crew walk-off. David had become very sick and Joe was afraid he would never see him again if he didn't get to go to the party. So on the evening of the party I spirited Joe out of the hospital and into a cab and to Manhattan Plaza, where the party was held. We spent a couple of hours there, and Joe sat a while with David, who was very thin and miserable. It was spiritually deflating for Joe to see David, who had been so handsome, withered away to nothing, sitting in a wheelchair with a lot of people who had essentially come to say good-bye.

By time we got back to the hospital, Joe was depressed and angry. I got him in the room and had just hung up his jacket when a voice behind me said, "Just where have you two been?" I turned around and saw a nurse, not looking very amused, standing in the doorway like a bouncer at the Saint. This brought back every brush with authority I ever had—nuns, principals, teachers, cops. I almost wet my pants. I don't know what I was afraid of—what could she do, throw us out? Have me arrested for kidnapping? "Well," she said in a tone that said that she absolutely had to be someone's mother, "where have you two been?"

I really wish I could lie. I've never been any kind of liar, and Joe, for all his acting aspirations, was worse. It was good then that I couldn't think of anything to say, because anything I would have said would have only been absurd. Joe made the effort.

"We were in the cafeteria—chatting," he said. I looked at him in awe. It sounded so lame the way he said it.

"The cafeteria is closed," she said in a way that challenged Joe into an attitude.

"We were chatting," he said, "not eating. We needed to have a talk." He was beginning to sound convincing.

"Well, next time you boys need to go to the cafeteria, let us know at the nurses' station. Everyone was looking for you. You had us scared."

She left and shut the door. I giggled for some ridiculous reason, feeling guilty. It was that last little bit about us putting them out, I suppose. It never takes much. But Joe just slumped down in his bed with images of a frail and barely living David haunting him in a way you could see in his eyes. I lay down in my cot next to his bed, and we held hands through the side until we fell asleep.

After getting out of the hospital Joe began to lose weight, and a few new Kaposi's sarcoma lesions appeared on his body. Some of the old ones became raised and angry looking. But the most troubling thing was that he was never quite able to get his breath back. Then after a series of tests we got the news that the Kaposi's sarcoma had entered Joe's lungs. He had lung cancer. We took the news in stride and kept waking up each day, recognizing that things were fragile but trying to appreciate the time we had.

We had a small dinner party on Thanksgiving with Jane and Griffin Gold as guests. I roasted a goose, which I had never done before but which turned out superbly. An Englishman named Kevin, who was the GMHC volunteer coordinator and who would die the following year, gave me the secret to roasting perfect goose. We all felt pretty Dickensian and special. Jane took photographs, and the dinner was fun. The only dark spot was that Joe had had to say good-bye to two friends that day who were leaving to go home for a while. Michael Calvert, a fellow PWAC member, was going home to Georgia for a stay of undetermined length. Joe also had a friend, Tony, who didn't have AIDS, who was leaving for northern Wisconsin. I had met Tony while Joe was in the hospital. He was probably an old boyfriend of Joe's because he was extremely handsome with what I call cappuccino looks—dark, rich, and roasted. Like Joe, he had those actor-model-waiter features, and he was very down to earth. He was a great help while Joe was in the hospital, and I looked to him with some hope for the future that after Joe died,

I would have Tony as the one friend of Joe's who was not sick. He was the only well friend Joe had. When Joe had to say good-bye to them both on the same day over Thanksgiving weekend, he came into the house dark and somber. He didn't think that he'd ever see either of them again, and he cried. He knew if he got another bout of pneumocystis, he would be unlikely to survive it. Knowing he would probably be feeling this way, I went out that morning and bought him a few gifts to cheer him up. The first gift was a book of *Far Side* cartoons, which he loved, and the second was a miniature crystal red rose in a vase, no higher than three inches. That day, the presents worked and cheered him up. He came in from saying good-bye separately to Michael and Tony. He looked at the coffee table where there were two neatly wrapped gifts.

"What are those?" he asked.

"Presents," I said.

"For me?" he said, like he was 10 years old.

"Yep." He smiled and opened them, and we had a happy afternoon. Later, when he went into the hospital again, he took the little crystal rose with him.

### SPENDING ALL MY MONEY IN TIFFANY'S

The three best months of the year in New York are May, because the weather is so wonderful; October because of the leaves; and December, because of Christmas. We had decided to spend Christmas in New York, and I was determined to make it a special one. Early in December, his mother, who rarely called and when she did she was more inclined to talk about herself than him, visited us with his two sisters, who were great. I guess no one really likes his mother-in-law, and if that is so, I can't be counted as an exception. During their visit I tried, but she always made me feel like an outsider in my own home. She didn't ask what she could do to help us. It just reinforced the notion that had taken root in my own mentality—we could count on only ourselves. After their visit we spent Christmas itself together alone. It had always been the tradition in my family that each person gets a series of gifts, which are opened progressively, leading up to the main present, which is the climax. I followed that tradition with Joe.

For his crowning-glory Christmas present I went shopping at Tiffany's. I wasn't earning much money at GMHC, and Joe wasn't working. Not all of Joe's medications were covered by Medicaid or by insurance, and so they had to be paid for out of pocket. Money was tight. But I walked into Tiffany's and took a big chance in buying Joe a gold wedding band. We had never talked about this part of relationships, and I didn't know how he would feel about having one. But I did know how I felt about giving him one. It was a cold and very cloudy day, with winds carrying snatches of snow when I walked across Central Park to Fifth Avenue, marched into Tiffany's, and walked around for a bit as if I knew what I was doing. I glanced from counter to counter, afraid that someone was going to ask me to leave. I didn't feel I could ask anyone where they were. "Are you getting married?" they would ask. No, I just feel like buying one. I sauntered from counter to counter, gathering my intelligence. Finally, I was able to determine where they were, and I walked up to the counter where I saw wedding bands.

The salesman was a young 24-year-old who sounded Texan by his accent. He was over six feet tall with well-cut blond hair, wearing a double-breasted blue jacket. He had straight white teeth and was startlingly handsome.

"May I help you?" I jumped out of my skin. I was self-conscious enough to interpret this less as an inquiry and more as a challenge to buy something.

"I wanted to look at these…wedding bands." I pointed at them quickly, as if I were afraid they'd jump up and bite me if I got too close. He reached in and took out the velvety trays of wedding bands. My stomach knotted, wondering how many billions of dollars this was going to cost. I wondered if he wondered what a man was doing looking at men's wedding bands. He carefully brought a tray out and put them on the counter. I wondered if I had lost my mind. You would think I was planning a heist rather than a legitimate purchase. I began trying several on but focused on one that was a little too large for me and looked as if it were three rings fused together to make one. I tried to discreetly discern the price.

"I'll take this," I said, shy but trying to be sophisticated, as though I didn't care I was spending the last $500 I had. He smiled.

"Excellent choice." They must practice that line. "Will you be presentin' this to a gentleman friend as a gift for Christmas," said the salesman in a most professional Southern manner, inclining his head to me ever so slightly as he asked the question. I was so surprised I gave him my very best smile.

"Why, yes, as a matter of fact, I will," wanting to add a little "fiddleedee" at the end.

"Well, then," he said, "would you like me to have it gift-wrapped?"

"No, no," I said, "I think I'd like to do that myself." He smiled. I will always be Tiffany's biggest fan.

---

*28,275 new cases of AIDS were diagnosed*
*16,013 more people died*
*A cumulative total of 69,363 cases were diagnosed*
*40,221 people were dead of AIDS in America*

---

## THE EXPECTED AND THE UNEXPECTED

The ring was a big hit. Christmas was so wonderful, and we both got a gift when my landlord called to give us word that we were moving into a new and bigger apartment upstairs. Up to that time we had been living in a studio on the ground floor of a great building at 75th Street and Broadway. It was a large studio but a studio nonetheless. As it turned out, they had decided to create an office in that space and would move us to a one-bedroom on the seventh floor. Only a few days before the call, Joe and I were talking as we lay in bed late at night. "Honey," he said, "do you think we could get a one-bedroom apartment?"

"I don't see how," I said. "You're not working, and it feels like we can barely afford this one. Besides it would be a monumental task to find one."

We called the landlord's call Miracle on 75th Street.

Then a few days into the new year, we met with sudden disaster. It was an example of how fragile a PWA's existence is. Michael Calvert was very sick in Georgia. Tony was still in Wisconsin and was going to be staying there the entire winter. I had been out doing some shopping for Joe's birthday, which was coming up on the twelfth of January. When I got home the house was quiet. I walked into the living room to find that Grif was there with Joe. They both sat there, saying nothing.

I knew by the looks on their faces that Michael Calvert must have died. I put down my packages. No one said anything. Grif looked sick. Joe looked blank. "Is Michael OK?" I asked quietly.

"Tony," said Joe.

"What about Tony?"

"Tony is dead."

It took me a moment to try to figure out what he meant. Michael was sick; Tony was fine.

"How can Tony be dead?"

"He killed himself in his garage in Wisconsin. He was depressed, he got drunk, and he killed himself. Carbon monoxide."

In the wake of the shock it was quiet for a moment while a number of feelings came to the surface. I felt so much anger and so much betrayal. And if I felt that way, I couldn't imagine what Joe must have felt. I had grown accustomed to the fact that Tony would be there for me after Joe died. He had his health. He was blessed with good looks. He had so many things going for him. Poor Michael was sick and dying and fighting for his life, and then Tony just up and throws it all away. He wasted it all. It was such a stunning thought it was difficult to take in. Joe sat there, staring. Each of my attempts at comfort seemed to fall flat and meaningless.

Grif suggested that they go for a walk and get something to eat. I was relieved when they left. Their sorrow felt so oppressive, and I was so angry. I cleaned up around the house, muttering to myself about Tony's betrayal. The telephone rang. I answered to hear the news from his mother that Michael Calvert died that morning. Joe was going to have to say good-bye to them both again on the same day.

At that moment I would have rather been almost anyone else on earth I could imagine. Outside our front door was a fruit and flower stand. I went outside and bought a red rose and put it into a crystal vase on the coffee table. I sat on the couch and waited for Joe to come home. Telling him what had happened was one of the most difficult things I have ever had to do.

When Joe came home he was obviously feeling better. Grif had gone home. I took his coat and kissed him hello. He looked at the coffee table.

"You got a rose," he said.

"Yep, I did. Do you remember that day when Michael and Tony both left town and I brought you the little crystal rose?"

"Sure."

"Well, Joe, that's why I went out and bought this one." He looked at me and back at the rose and then back at me. "Michael Calvert died this morning." He slipped his arms around me, and I held him for a long time while he cried.

Joe entered a deep depression after his birthday that lasted for days. It was so bad that he wouldn't respond to direct questions from me. If I asked him what he wanted for dinner, he wouldn't reply. If I said I was going to the store, he'd get his jacket and go with me but wouldn't say a word. He wouldn't speak but would eat. After a week it was over, and he recovered. But the week had been like living with someone who was in a coma. At times it was so oppressive that all life in the apartment was stifled. Whatever room he was in I would leave, just to get away from that overwhelming presence of grief. He emerged from it almost as suddenly and dramatically as the news of the deaths of Michael and Tony had reached us. Somehow he returned to his world of trying to survive despite all the mounting evidence to the contrary.

Not long after we moved upstairs. My mother flew out to help us. I had been rather worried about that. She had never met a boyfriend of mine, nor had she ever met anyone with AIDS before. Joe was so sensitive just now that if she inadvertently said the wrong thing, it could provoke a strong reaction from him. Or he could just end up shutting down again. But when she arrived, she had brought us both crew neck sweaters that were alike, which we both thought very cute of her. My mother was very charming. You would have thought that she met people with AIDS every day. She had certainly come a long way in a short time from the day she expressed her fear I would get AIDS from writing Paul's will. She and Joe would talk for long periods of time, usually out of range of my hearing. They liked to tease me that they were talking about me. I'm sure they were. I realized that I was no longer so sure which was my greatest fear—that they wouldn't like each other or that they would like each other and share secrets. Every time I heard them laugh, I froze with apprehension just as I did when I heard my mother utter the words "When Mark was little…" and then I couldn't hear anymore.

Despite the deaths of Michael and Tony, with my mother there and the new apartment, it felt like we were getting the year off with things going our way, even if our friends didn't fare so well. I had to look for hope where I could get it.

## IS THIS KS?

One day at work as I was walking to my office, Kevin, the Englishman who had supplied me with the excellent method of roasting a goose, stopped me.

"Darling, could you come into my office for a moment?" he asked.

"Sure."

We went in and he sat at his desk.

"Forgive me for this darling," he said. He looked ever-so-much like Roddy McDowell. "I'm sure people do this sort of thing to you all the time, but I figure since you live with Joe, you could tell me about this."

I wasn't following him. He shut the door to his office and began to unbutton his shirt. I still did not know what the hell was going on. Once undone all the way, he pulled open his shirt to reveal his right pectoral.

"Is this KS?" he asked. We had all been through this so many times. Gay doctors were very busy answering this question about bruises and scrapes and dermatological normalities often. We asked each other these questions all the time, and the response was usually, "No. No way. That isn't KS. You are being ridiculous—it's a bruise, silly. Look at the green around the edge. It's just a bruise."

But I looked at Kevin's lesion and knew immediately that it was KS. There was no question at all in my mind. Kevin was right; in living with Joe, I was able to spot KS in a second. There were times on the subway when I would examine marks on my fellow passengers, now and then finding a K.S. lesion on the back of someone's neck, and wonder if they knew about it yet.

What could I say to Kevin? As sure as I was, I wasn't about to go out on a limb and tell him he had it. "Well," I said, "you know, Kevin, I think that you would be real justified in calling your doctor right away and asking him to biopsy that for you."

"So you think it is?"

"I think it is worth finding out."

His soft-brown eyes looked at my face for an answer. I was determined to give him none. Kevin found out he did have KS. He asked me to do his will, and he died not long afterward. My friend Rick Croll took his place as volunteer coordinator. That was often the way promotions came about at GMHC.

## MAGIC BULLETS

Then came a ray of hope. We had always looked desperately for something to hang on to. The epidemic was still so young and science and medicine, after all, had always been so virile in the face of challenge. Polio and smallpox had been picked off. We put a man on the moon. Tuberculosis was, then at least, under control. AIDS was the first significant challenge to modern medicine in the second half of the 20th century. If we had

had money to bet, we would have put it on science. Surely a cure would be found. Of that there was no question. The only question was one of time. Would we have the time?

I used to lie awake at night, holding Joe and wondering when my Superman image of science would fly through the window. My original assessment of the epidemic when Todd first read about it to me hasn't changed. It was, I thought, going to take at least 20 years. But I'd been wrong before; maybe I would be again. I had sort of gotten my hopes up when Rock Hudson flew to Paris on a stretcher, but those hopes quickly dried up and blew away with the hard wind of reality. But just maybe something else would come along. There it would appear in the headlines: MIRACLE CURE FOR AIDS. Joe would take it, and I would have him with me for years and years, and the pain of the epidemic would have paid off in the end as we realized how much we loved each other and how important it was that we do love each other. As we realized that we are stronger than we ever thought we were. As we understood that deep inside us there is enough of God to make miracles happen. And so I lay there at night holding Joe's hand—and my breath—and I waited.

And then in March it came. The magic bullet. It was an old form of chemotherapy that had been tried and failed, but it appeared in the test tube to inhibit the replication of the virus. We called our doctor. We had to have it. And in what seemed a miraculously short though tense time, we did have it. It couldn't have come soon enough. It was called AZT.

Now, AZT was a curious thing. It appeared like a fast train out of the night. One minute it is quiet, and the next minute it is coming down the tracks with the force and speed that was unimaginable. And like a train, it was just about as expensive, costing $10,000 for a one-year supply. Burroughs Wellcome, the drug's manufacturer, would keep it at that price until the fall of 1989, when it would bow to pressure from the community and lower the cost by 20%. The drug had been developed years before for other purposes with research money largely rumored to have been provided in large part by our tax dollars. Nevertheless, Burroughs Wellcome began charging the astronomical sum of $800 per month for a prescription. It was the most expensive prescriptive drug in history.

There was nothing I wouldn't do to pay it. I would have opened lines of credit, borrowed from my family, or stolen money to pay for AZT, a drug made from the sperm of a particular fish. That supposedly added to the cost. And I had been charging some of Joe's drugs on my already overburdened MasterCard.

Little capsules filled with medicine on the inside, filled with hope on the outside. The hope we attached to those capsules was very powerful. We looked at them in awe as if they were manna from heaven. Little pills made from the sperm of a fish. That seemed the funniest and most ironic of all. When we got the capsules, we took them home and went into our bedroom. I gave Joe a tall glass of water. He sat on the floor of the bedroom with capsules in hand. We examined them in our hands as if they were visiting creatures from outer space. Joe held out the first two blue-and-white capsules. It was an attractively designed capsule, I thought; they know their audience. It was like a designer capsule.

"Well," he said, "it was sperm that got me into this mess, and it's gonna be sperm that gets me out, I suppose." He raised his cupped hand to his lips and swallowed the glass of water. I said a prayer. I always pray to the Virgin Mary because I feel as if I can trust her, since the rest of them are men.

The next morning, I asked him how he felt, not really expecting that he would tell me that he already felt better.

"Not so good," he said.

We waited.

A week later Joe's joints all hurt and he felt fluish. As it turned out, the doctor cited this as a possible side effect. An additional side effect was that anemia was certainly possible.

But nothing happened with the AZT. There was no real difference in Joe from before, except that he seemed to be losing more and more weight. Before getting sick, he had weighed 185 pounds. He had lost some weight after getting pneumocystis, but when he started taking the AZT, he lost even more and his weight dropped to 162. Then he became anemic.

It became even more frustrating when the anemia set in. At that time the daily dosage for AZT was much higher than it is now. The anemia, therefore, presented itself sooner and more strongly. Instead of making him better, instead of erasing AIDS, the AZT was making him sicker. Yet, of course, we believed that it was like chemotherapy. He had to get sicker to get better. But his weight continued to drop, and he began to cough chronically.

I began to cook frantically. Anything to get him going again. I began to believe that my cooking and AZT combined could be our salvation. Throughout the length of this illness, like a Jewish mother, I believed in the power of my cooking. I began to make iron-rich foods—spinach and liver and onions. Joe would push it around his plate while I enthusiastically downed mine, covered with onions, spinach wilted in olive oil and garlic.

"They say," he said somewhat accusingly, "that the virus feeds on iron."

It made me feel like Benedict Arnold when he said that. Here I was making all of these iron-rich foods and it might be helping the virus I was trying to help defeat. That was the way it seemed so often. Every time I tried to help, it was the wrong thing.

"Oh, I see," I said without seeing. "Well, that's kind of frustrating, isn't it. What am I supposed to make then?"

Joe didn't answer. He just pushed his food around on his plate. The magic bullet had missed its target by a mile.

It was as though he were on a gentle slope through the winter and into the spring. He had more and more trouble breathing. There was no lovemaking, though we fell asleep every night holding hands and talking, telling each other how we felt, making wishes, and playing pretend. One night we both recited poems we had memorized while we held hands. The soft touch of his hand and the quiet lilt of his voice in the dark saying the poetry of T.S. Eliot is one of the most romantic memories I have. We made almost weekly desperate trips to the doctor. He had developed a serious cough that increased in severity but never went away. The cough was horrible at times, a cold and sharp cough that tells the listener there is more wrong than can be cured.

His doctor could not diagnose it, but nevertheless blindly prescribed all sorts of drugs. His next doctor was someone neither of us fully trusted, a feeling that had seemed confirmed when we first got Joe's AZT. It had been promised and delayed several times. We really wanted it; it stood between us and death, we were certain. You can't imagine the longing we felt. Finally the doctor said Joe's prescription had arrived, but when we got it and examined the bottle, we could see that the prescription label was pasted over another prescription label. The AZT had belonged to someone else, someone who had presumably died. Joe was furious.

Then he began to enter a really bad time. We had to order an oxygen tank for the bedside. He could not eat unless he lay down in bed on his belly; it was the only way he could eat and still breath. He looked pathetic lying facedown on the bed, eating his food. The lesion on his forehead became more pronounced. The one on his thigh was tall and angry. As the AZT made him more anemic, his energy level reached a new low. His smooth and beautiful skin became dry, and I applied bottles of moisturizer to him every week.

I made food look as attractive as possible, but he lost his appetite. The weight began to fall off his large frame. During the time we had been together, he went from 180 pounds to 130. He began to have digestive failure all the time. It would be really embarrassing for him on the street when he would throw up and I would hold him and people passed by, politely not noticing but noticing all the same. That really is the nice thing about New Yorkers—an attitude often misperceived by out-of-towners as "coldness" is really very polite deference. But after an episode of throwing up on the street, Joe would be embarrassed and sometimes cry and push me away.

Then there was a new magic bullet. It was out of Israel and called AL721. I didn't realize at the time that we were falling into a cruel pattern that would resonate the rest of the epidemic. Already there had been cyclosporin, ribavirin, and others. Joe had already made one junket to Mexico to buy ribavirin that was useless. Later, these magic bullets would take on different forms and originate from different countries. The bitter melon from the Philippines, an enema men with AIDS would give themselves; Compound Q, a cucumber root from China that would be injected into the veins of people with AIDS, causing seizures in some; the kombucha mushroom, used in Russia and which people could grow in their own kitchen and distill tea from that would provide miracle cures for everything. But back in 1986 it was AL721 for me. It was so easy, you could get instructions for mixing it in your own kitchen and then freezing it. Joe didn't like the taste and wouldn't eat it. I found that there were foods that would disguise the taste so I would sneak it into his food. My best hiding places were in mashed potatoes or oatmeal. He might grow suspicious and ask and I would look out the window and be quiet.

But for a while it went from bad to worse. One Friday we visited the doctor, who told us Joe's red-cell counts were extremely low. The anemia, he said, was critical, and he wanted Joe to go into the hospital. At this point Joe's cancer made it necessary for us to carry the portable oxygen unit with us to the doctor. Joe refused to go into the hospital. The doctor insisted. Joe still refused. The doctor turned to me and said that he wasn't going to take responsibility in that case. Responsibility for what, I asked? He then took me aside and said that Joe could very well die over the weekend and that I should be prepared for that. On our way home Joe asked me what the doctor had said. As I've said, I don't lie, so I told him.

It was a long weekend. I couldn't help but to believe that I would wake up with a dead person lying next to me after the doctor had said that. I begged him to go to the hospital for a transfusion, but he angrily refused. There were actually two times when I thought he was dead—once while he was taking a nap and once again in the morning after I awoke. I didn't want to try to wake him, so I put a mirror from my contact lens case under his nose. I felt silly doing this and knew that there would be certain hell to pay if he caught me, but I was terrified of losing him suddenly. I scrutinized his face for The Look. The doctor's warning echoed in the apartment for the entire weekend. At night I awoke every few hours to stare at him in the dark and see if he was alive. It was an elephant in the room that we pretended wasn't there at all.

He did not die during the weekend. When Monday morning came it was as though all danger was passed, though of course that wasn't so. But I was furious with the doctor for his attitude and putting me in the position of anxiety and utter helplessness. Still, I phoned home every few hours on some pretext, just to make sure that Joe was alive. I would space out the calls so that it wasn't too apparent what I was doing, and then I would make the last call at about 2:30 in the afternoon. Then when it was time for me to go home at 5:30 or 6, I would run from my office to the subway in Chelsea and then home from the subway station near our apartment, just to get home sooner to find out if he was all right and to be with him. I knew that there wasn't much time left for us.

## CLUB MED

I decided we should switch doctors. I thought that he should see an oncologist because of the infiltration of the cancer in his lungs. He had lung cancer, I reasoned, and so he should be seeing an oncologist, not a doctor who treated AIDS.

Joe agreed and we made an appointment with Dr. Linda Laubenstein at New York University Medical Center. Dr. Laubenstein was herself in a wheelchair, having had polio. She would become the inspiration for the doctor character in Larry Kramer's *The Normal Heart*.

The day of the appointment Joe was in very bad shape. He weighed only 130 pounds, and we had to take the portable oxygen unit. He was very weak, and getting him ready for the doctor took me hours. I had to get him up and get him fed in bed on his belly. Cleaning up that mess, I would draw a bath because it was the only way I could clean him, short of holding him up in the shower with me, which was dangerous because it was clumsy and difficult. Then I'd carry him into the bath and wash him like he was a big Ken doll. His head would lean over the side of the tub or against my chest. Then I'd dry him off and toss him back in bed while I took my shower. Then I'd get him dressed. Then I'd get myself dressed. Naturally, it was pissing rain, so I got our umbrellas and both our backpacks and our portable oxygen tank. We managed downstairs to get a cab in the rain, a miracle in and of itself. When we arrived at the doctor's office, Joe was exhausted and was leaning on me in the cab. I looked at the driver as we pulled up and could tell that, other than driving us there, he was going to be no help to me. So I paid him and then got out on my side and opened the door on the other side. I got the back packs, the useless umbrellas, the tank, and Joe and pulled everything out of the cab. I put both backpacks on one shoulder and the portable oxygen tank on my other shoulder. Then I picked Joe up and carried him through the pouring rain and into the medical center lobby. Fortunately for us both, there was a wheelchair nearby, and I threw him in it like a limp bag of wash. He sat in a pile with both backpacks and the tank on top of him. We were also a little damp from the rain. I dried us off and fixed his hair—he was still very particular about how he looked—and we made for the elevator.

We waited in the examination room, Joe slumped over in a chair. Dr. Laubenstein, who had been examining his X-rays, rolled into the room. She was a no-bullshit woman. She had some of his X-rays with her. She looked at Joe square in the eye. She said, "You are going to die."

Joe flinched. I flinched. She went on.

"It is just a matter of time. You have lung cancer, and you have it bad. We can maybe buy some time. It won't be easy. We will have to do chemotherapy. There may be side effects. You may lose your hair. You may be nauseous. Do you think you want to try it? Yes or no?"

We looked at each other. My face pleaded with him. Joe didn't hesitate. He said yes. I cannot honestly say that in his position I would have said that. Longevity has never really been my goal. I'm not sure what the benefits of longevity are. I am struck by the fact that we talk in the spiritual sense about a wonderful afterlife, but we fight like hell to keep from getting there. Is that instinct?

Dr. Laubenstein then wheeled around and began to create a magic potion. She got a long hypodermic and a few bottles and stuck the needle into each bottle withdrawing the elixir. That day she injected Joe with a mixture of two kinds of chemotherapy. We watched her turn the bottles upside down over a needle and mix a blend of clear substances and inject it into Joe's vein. This to me, was like watching Jesus turn water into wine. We watched it go in with hope, and as it disappeared from the syringe, I said a prayer. We went home and waited. That night in bed Joe told me that the only reason he was trying the chemotherapy was that he wanted for us to have more time together.

I began to think I was imagining things when I saw that within a few days the lesions seemed different to me. It sounds ridiculous, but they looked less angry, even cowed by the chemotherapy. I decided I was projecting. But then Joe began to walk around the apartment without his oxygen tank. He began to eat sitting up.

The following week, even Dr. Laubenstein was somewhat stunned when Joe walked into her office for his second appointment. He went to her office in a cab, unaccompanied. He left the portable oxygen unit at home. We had stopped using the bedside unit a few days before. He had color and energy. It was a fucking miracle, and it was so refreshing to learn that I could still believe in them.

He got better and better. I had become expert at cooking extremely fattening meals that looked like they had been a lot of trouble to prepare, when in fact they weren't all that much. But the appearance of trouble I knew would make him feel that he had to eat it. He ate them all and gained 23 pounds back over the next four weeks. The lesion on his forehead, which was the oldest lesion and which had grown quite angry, was now flat and opaque. His breathing was less difficult. He had energy. He began to look himself. The lesion on his thigh began to disappear with the regular doses of chemotherapy.

On Easter Sunday, however, we were reminded of how fragile he still was. We were going to church and were trying to get a cab. He was on one side of Broadway, and I was on the other—we would take a cab going in any direction. He got one first, and I began to walk to the corner to get across the street. As I did, a man walked up and began to get into the cab that Joe had hailed. Joe must have said something to him. Joe put his hand on the man's shoulder. The guy wheeled around, and there were words exchanged. I stood helpless across Broadway, so mad I could feel my pulse in my throat. Then I watched incredulously as the two began to shove each other. The man pushed Joe down on the curb and got into the cab and sped away. I got across Broadway and picked Joe up while he brushed his clothes. He was more excited than angry. He smiled and looked at me and said, "If I were still in my prime, we'd be in that cab now." He was only 32. But he was so much better already, maybe he would return to his prime.

But there was no question that things had taken a dramatic turn. Just the fact that we were going to church at all, or going anywhere, was amazing. I was so touched that God had truly answered my prayers. The magic bullet. Joe became a different person. The dreaded oxygen unit next to our bed, always a reminder of what was happening, sat unused. He no longer ate in bed lying on his belly but at the table with me. He was no longer unshaven and in a bathrobe but in clothes, looking like a regular person. If this was happening on the outside of his body, it stood to reason it must be happening on the inside. He was so alive again. And his appetite for food was not the only appetite to return. Lovemaking returned as a ferocious art form. I walked into work smiling a lot.

In response to increasing press there had been a steady increase in the number of volunteers we had in the department as AIDS gained more notoriety. What began as 15 or 20 people who met in various living rooms with Steve Gittleson was growing into an impressive number. And they came from all kinds of law firms. Many of the early volunteers were lawyers who had their own small practices and didn't have to necessarily fear the stigma of being associated with this work. But we began getting calls from managing partners and young associates who wanted to volunteer time. Large law firms began supplying both bodies and resources. This changed the nature of my job considerably. Not only was I less involved in the daily effort of visiting deathbeds because there were more volunteers, but the nature of the practice itself took on a wider and deeper value, meaning we were able to address insurance and discrimination matters as well as estate issues. I had not only more volunteers but a staff. An assistant, another assistant, and even another lawyer were hired. We even began to work on immigration problems, leaving me less in a hands-on role and more involved in strategizing and administering a growing law practice, though I still wrote an occasional deathbed will. In many respects this came along at an ideal time because it allowed me to spend more time on Joe and less time in hospitals with other people. It was espe-cially welcomed now that Joe seemed to be feeling better. It was also welcomed because it meant I had more resources to face deathbed-will situations—a scene I preferred to avoid just then. Each one was a reminder of what might come. Still, whenever Joe went into the hospital, I would get a list of clients who were patients who had requested wills and visit them while I was stay-ing with Joe. Those were never easy. In a way I began to feel like a patient myself. When Joe got better, I was better.

There were a few setbacks, though. A few weeks after gaining strength, Joe experienced some headaches that wouldn't go away. He had to be checked out during a hospital visit that would last a few days and that would include a spinal tap. We were put into a section of New York University hospital called Co-op Care, which is a dramatically good idea both emotional-ly and economically. It is a section of the hospital carved out to be less hospital-like and more hotel-like. Tests and procedures are run in a centrally located medical portion on one lower floor, while patients are admitted to the upper floors. The real factor that makes the difference is that on the upper patient floors, there are no nurses' stations. Taking the place of nurses is the pa-tient's care partner—his spouse, his friend, his relative, his lover. Care of the patient was left to the care partner, who took care of the room, served the meals (or you could go together to the main dining room), got the linens, took the vital signs, and called them into the central nurses' station below. Some of the rooms were actually suites, where there was a sitting room, separate and apart from a bedroom, though most of the units were just single rooms with two beds and amenities. Even though we had never had a suite, we loved it here because we got to stay together privately, and we knew that care was only a moment away. But it did not feel like being in the hospital, and the cost per day was a fraction of what a regular hospital stay would be. Walking the wide hallways, the only way you would know you were in a hospital would be by noting the railings attached to all the hallway walls to help people with their stability. Otherwise, it looked like you might be aboard a ship, a fact reinforced that by the fact that the population seemed overwhelmingly made up of elderly couples. Now with the AIDS crisis in full swing, there were a growing number of same-sex male couples. The popular name for Co-op Care was Club Med, and we loved it because in many ways it really was like a vacation.

When the time came I took Joe to the medical procedure area, where he would have his spinal tap, the thought of which was making me queasy. I had seen a lot of medical procedures and dying people in my time at GMHC, but the thought of a spinal tap put me to the test. When we got downstairs, the doctor asked me if I was going to want to stay in the room.

I opted to wait outside, and when Joe came out, he said that it hadn't been too bad and that he felt fine. I pushed him in his wheelchair back to our room. We were given instructions that he should remain perfectly still, since the tap could cause a severe headache if he moved around much. Apparently, since he felt so fine afterward, he didn't take this too seriously and that night he slipped out of his bed and came into mine in quite a frisky mood. I warned him again about movement, but he didn't listen. The next morning he had a massive headache.

I had to take him for X-rays. I wasn't very good at the wheel-

chair navigation yet. It is easy for a person pushing to assume
that the person riding is fine, as long as you aren't running into
walls. As I was pushing him across the courtyard, Joe leaned over
the side and vomited. He was embarrassed by this, and he yelled
at me that I was pushing too fast. It was one of those moments
when I realized how vulnerable he was and how much he must
resent having so little control over what was going on in his life.
There was a virus eating away his immune system, he was dying,
people treated him differently, his whole life had been disrupted, and virtually everything from the state of his immune system
to the way he felt from one moment to the next to his very navigation was beyond his control and authority. When he yelled at
me I could hear not just irritation but anguish and anger at me
who could be so much in control. Feeding him, giving his medication, doing his laundry, bathing him like he was a big doll.
Control is a big issue for people with life-threatening illnesses,
and I understood that well in the course of my work with people with AIDS, but rarely did it appear so apparent to me as it
did that spring day on the square in front of the hospital next to
a puddle of vomit.

## AN UNEXPECTED VISIT

Being in Club Med was a good, safe feeling, but it is a lot of
work for the care partner. In addition to taking care of Joe I had
to continue going to work, which was located downtown on
the west side. The hospital was midtown on the east side, and our
apartment was on the upper west side. I would arrange for people to drop in on him during the day to make sure that all was

well and that he didn't get too bored. I would have to run home to collect the mail and feed our two cats, Rupert and Ginger Pye, and then take a cab back down and across town to the hospital. One day while I was at work Joe called with auspicious news. "Guess who's joining us for dinner?"

I was busy and not in the best of moods, feeling fairly overwhelmed by my schedule, which included trips to other hospitals to see clients. "Who?" I asked flatly.

"My mother," he said. I could hear him smiling. For some sadistic reason, he seemed amused.

At the risk of repeating myself, I have to say I really didn't care for this woman. After her Christmas visit, during which I tried my best by installing a large tree into the apartment and cooking a capon for her dinner to show her that we were a nice and normal household, she had some religious organization begin sending us Jesus tracts through the mail. The real clincher came when I received a bill for the tracts. It was not like we weren't hurting for money. I was supporting us on a pretty meager salary, what my mother provided from time to time, and Joe got social security. She had never asked us if we needed help. And with this she seemed to presume that we were sinners in need of saving. This despite the fact that I was the one caring for her son while she sat a thousand miles away tossing an occasional phone call his way. I could not figure out what in this scenario made her think she was acting in a Christian manner. But that's who she was, and the idea of trying to change her outlook struck me as futile. When the bill for the Jesus tracts arrived, I firmly told Joe that he had better call her and tell her we weren't paying for them, and he heard the no-nonsense tone in my voice. I don't know what their conversation was like, but the tracts stopped. Her husband worked for an airline, and she could visit us any time she wanted free of charge, a frightening prospect for a mother-in-law.

"She's not staying with us, is she?" I asked.

"No," he said, "she's flying in this morning and out tonight. She is just going to eat dinner."

"Do you want to be alone with her?" I asked pleadingly. "I mean, I don't mind grabbing a bite elsewhere so you two can spend some time together."

"No," he said, crushing all my hopes and enjoying it, "we'll have the whole afternoon together, and she will want to ask you questions."

I was broken-hearted. I got to the hospital as soon as I could after work, and there she was with Joe in the cafeteria at Club Med. We had a polite dinner, though she didn't ask any burning questions and thankfully it came time for her to go the airport rather quickly. She kissed Joe good-bye, and I offered to go downstairs and help her catch a cab. When we got down to the street, a cab mercifully came up before long. As she was stepping into it, without having ever thanked me for anything I had done and still without asking if we needed any help, she stuck a short finger up in the air and into my face and said, "Now you take good care of my son."

She shut the door and drove off. "Well, I will." I said to her fading taillights. "Someone has got to do it."

It was the last time she saw Joe. After he died, she never called me to see how I was doing. I guess she didn't like me either.

## ANNIVERSARY

We had actually gone out on our first date on April 12, the date we regarded as our anniversary. Joe was well enough after only a few weeks on the chemo to want to go out. It was a very rainy spring night, and we went down to a small restaurant in the Village; it was the kind of place where there are only four or five tables. The food was fantastic. They didn't serve alcohol, but you could take your own, and so we took along a good bottle of our favorite champagne. The waitress brought us their two best champagne glasses—flutes trimmed in gold. We also had an appetizer.

Even though it was a small place, it seemed very private, the other couples sitting at their tables absorbed in their own lives. Joe took out his key ring and set it on the table. He had one of those silver Tiffany key rings, and for some reason even though I will be forever a Tiffany slave, I did not like those key rings. On the other hand, I had a particularly distasteful key ring that was large and round like a jailer's, and Joe had always hated it. He asked me to put my key ring on the table. With some difficulty I pulled it out and set it down. He took it from me and removed each and every key and then asked me what that key was for. I knew what this was leading up to. I knew that it meant that he was giving me one of those tasteful Tiffany key rings like he had even though I didn't want it. And that was going to be my anniversary present? How romantic is a key ring? My heart sank. I thought to myself, *This is just like birthdays—it pays not to get too built up beforehand; otherwise, you are just disappointed. A key ring for my anniversary.*

We finished the recital of each key, of which there were many, and then Joe smiled, making those deep creases on both sides of those lips. He shoved all the keys back to my side of the table. Sitting in the middle of the pile was a Tiffany's wrapped box. I looked at it trying to feign excitement. A key ring.

I oohed and aahed over the blue box with the white ribbon. Slowly I opened it, concentrating on my expression so that I would appear surprised and pleased. I *was* surprised when I opened it because there was the ring I had given him for Christmas. I didn't know what it meant. Why was he giving me the ring back?

And then I looked at his hand; his ring was on his hand. I looked in the box, and there was the same ring. He told me that he had walked to Tiffany's from the apartment and gotten it with his sister when she had visited just a few days before. I put the ring on, still trying to catch up to the program. He had bought an identical ring except that mine was three colors of gold fused into one ring. I wondered if the same handsome Texan had helped him in Tiffany's.

"Well, aren't you goin' to kiss him?" shouted the next table. I reached over, and we kissed and we kissed and we kissed. The straight couple next to us raised their glasses in a toast and smiled. It was a cool and rainy night.

After he died I wore his ring on top of mine for a long time. Together, they look like one gold band. A few years later my friend Mike urged me to remove them. So I tried to take the two rings off every now and then, but I'm never able to keep them off my finger for more than a few months. I wish that weren't so, but it is.

## LIFE BECOMES NORMAL

We began to go out to dinner again, and even started going to the theater. That winter I had bought tickets for a performance of *Les Misérables* as soon as they went on sale. When he looked at the tickets, which were for a May performance, he told me that I shouldn't have wasted my money because he would never be able to go. We went to the show, and then we went to dinner at the restaurant that fired him for having AIDS. We ate a big dinner, and friends he had worked with came out to say hello. It was a very important night for Joe, to show them that he was still alive. It was a very important night for me because he was still alive.

Joe had gained almost 33 pounds. He was up to 163 and looked great. He no longer shuffled when he walked. My hope returned, and though I still ran home from the subway, it wasn't to see if he was alive. It was just to see him. His strength returned to the point where when PWAC called him to do a photo shoot for a poster for the Long Island AIDS Action Committee, Joe said he'd do it. It was a great feeling for him to have a job where he felt handsome and alive and more like Joseph the actor-model-waiter than Joseph the AIDS patient. Because we were both excited about it, I went with him to the photo shoot down in SoHo with a photographer named Janet Beller.

The shoot lasted almost four hours. There were several different poses and changes of clothes. I was amused to see that he had taken mostly clothes of mine for the shoot. He managed several different poses while Janet Beller stayed under a huge black cloth, her eye working the camera. I stood in back of her and from time to time whispered.

"Joe, pull up your sock, honey."

"Joe, lean this way."

"Joe, honey, your hair. Good."

Finally, Janet pulled the cloth from over her back.

"Hey, stage mom, come here," she said, looking at me. I was afraid I'd become too much interference and was now going to get the boot from the studio. I was prepared to beg to stay and promise I would behave when she said, "Go sit next to him. I want to take your picture together."

For the next half hour she shot the two of us. I remember as we sat there with this head resting gently against my cheek, I put my arm around him and vowed to myself that we would never get off this road now that we had found it. I was convinced absolutely that there was nothing we could not do together and that as long as I had breath in my body, I could protect Joe. My hope was so strong, I felt arrogant when it came to AIDS. After the shoot we went out for a romantic dinner and home for a romantic evening. We talked about plans to relocate to Los Angeles and start life up anew. The only thing that made us nervous was the thought of leaving Linda Laubenstein.

A few weeks later Janet Beller came by the apartment with a print for us of a photo she had taken. We both loved it. I felt like we looked very much in love.

On the last Sunday in May we went out to dinner in the neighborhood. It was cool and we both wore jackets. We had a very nice dinner together, and Joe was feeling very romantic. I asked him if he wanted to go somewhere for dessert, and he told me he wanted to only go home and get in bed and tell me how much he loved me. And since I was all for that, we did just that.

But when we were undressing for bed, he commented on how cold it was in the room. I shut the windows, but he began to shiver. I covered him with blankets when the convulsions started. He was not having a seizure; he was just so cold that he was out of control, with teeth chattering and his whole body shaking trying to get warm. I covered him with all the blankets we had, and it seemed to do no good. I took off all my clothes and got under the covers and laid on top of him to keep him warm. He held on to me with his arms and legs as if I were a life preserver. He didn't feel cold to me. In fact, all the blankets and his shivering heat put us at opposite ends of the spectrum. I could barely stand it because it was so hot, and he wouldn't let go. We stayed like that for about 15 or 20 minutes, when the polarity began to reverse. He felt normal for a bit, and then the fever started. I got out the thermometer and monitored him, and he went up to 104. He was so hot, we stripped off the blankets, and I got a pail of rubbing alcohol and immersed a wash cloth and bathed him all over his body with it. The alcohol seemed to immediately vaporize when it was washed onto his skin and steam that came off the washcloth was choking me. He was searing. Then he reversed again and became chilled. Again I lay down on top of him with all the blankets we owned, and I held him. The situation switched that way all night long. In the morning things settled down, and we both slept for a few hours. We got up, and I called Linda Laubenstein's office, but she was out of town at a conference. We packed up bags and headed across town to the hospital. That began the longest week of my life.

In the cab on the way over as we drove through Central Park, Joe was looking out the window on his side of the car.

"Does your church do gay marriages?" he asked. For the past few years, I had gone to Riverside Church, a very large multi-denominational church with a congregation of a few thousand on the upper west side. Joe had never expressed an interest in church, and certainly we had never talked about gay marriages.

"Yeah, it does. There's something called a ceremony of holy union or something like that," I said. "I've never been to one."

He didn't reply, he only nodded and looked out the window. I would never get to know what he was thinking about.

When we checked into the hospital, we were put in Club Med. This surprised me, since Joe seemed so bad, but apparently, there wasn't a great deal of choice given that hospital beds were scarce. Over the course of the next few days, I tended to Joe as best I could, but he seemed to be deteriorating rapidly. He was having a great deal of trouble breathing. They brought in a portable oxygen unit, but it proved to be insufficient. At night he was so bad, I became afraid that he would die right there in Club Med. It was obvious that our being there was medically in-appropriate. The physicians agreed, saying that Joe should go to the intensive care unit, but that there was no space there for him.

NYU Medical Center is shaped like a big *U*. Club Med is lo-cated in one wing, and in the opposing wing near the top is the intensive care unit. That night I sat in our room and looked across the expanse of the forecourt to the intensive care floor and prayed with one of the most unusual prayers I have ever made. While Joe fought for breath in his bed in the next room, I asked God to either make someone get well and leave the ICU or make someone get worse and take them away so that we could have their space. Heal them, God, or kill them. Your choice. But we have to get into the ICU.

I'll never know which happened, but we got transferred to ICU the next day. Joe was placed on a wall oxygen unit, which improved his blood gases somewhat but lacked any miraculous turnaround effect. Most frustrating was their inability to discover what was wrong. They could not isolate any particular kind of pneumonia. They began a wide-spectrum antibiotic. Antibiotics were always such a reliable fallback. Antibiotics always worked when I was a child. Surely a strong wide-spectrum antibiotic would do the trick. Surely we would get to go back to that interrupted romantic evening when we left the restaurant Sunday night.

But it didn't work. The blood gases got worse. And the worst was yet to come. When Joe was moved into intensive care, apparently it was policy that he receive an arterial catheter. This procedure involved the insertion of an obscenely long needle shoved up the groin. When they came in to perform the procedure, Joe was extremely frightened. He knew that he might be dying and his breathing was extremely distressed.

The doctor asked me to leave the room while the needles were being unwrapped and laid out. Joe insisted that I stay. I watched with some combination of nausea and fascination as the six-inch needle was placed next to Joe's scrotum and inserted. It was very much as if he had been stabbed. He screamed and blood ran all over the bed. I stood with weak knees, helpless, holding his hand and offering bleating words of useless encouragement. The procedure didn't take. They pulled the needle out.

The second time the doctor snapped at me to hold down Joe's

arms. He blamed Joe for the failure of the catheter to take hold. I looked at Joe. He was wet everywhere with sweat and tears. I grabbed both of his wrists and told him to look at the ceiling. The doctor unwrapped another needle, lifted Joe's nightshirt and inserted it. Joe bucked, and I held him down with all my strength. As he screamed, I felt an accomplice in his pain. I leaned down to his face and repeated over and over again, "I love you very much." We had placed our faith in this doctor we did not know, and I began to doubt that we had done the right thing. Again the procedure didn't take.

The third time I laid the upper part of my body on the upper part of Joe's. He held me and put his face in the small of my neck. When the third needle went into him, he screamed and screamed and screamed as badly as he had the first time. The third attempt failed. The room was crowded with the doctor and some nondescript personnel, all of whom were suited up—capped and gowned. Needless to say, I had given up on all that long ago.

"Don't let them do it anymore," pleaded Joe. "Don't let them do it."

"Remind me why we are doing this," I said.

"To monitor his vitals," said the doctor.

"Can't you just put a finger monitor on him?"

"No," replied the doctor.

"Why not?" I asked.

The only answer I remember getting was the equivalent of "because." He began to unwrap another needle.

"Well," I said, "we're not going to do this anymore."

"What?" said the doctor.

"I said, we're not going to do this anymore. You're not doing this again. You've tried, and it hasn't worked. We're using a finger monitor."

Over his mask, the doctor looked me in the eyes. He was sweating every bit as much as Joe and I were. "I'm the best there is," he actually said. "If I can't do this, no one can." I was struck even then that the doctor thought that this comment was remotely relevant.

"Then," I replied, "I guess no one is going to do it."

"I'm his doctor."

"Well, I'm his significant other, his power of attorney, and his lawyer." The doctor left the room, the obscene needles cleared away, the blood cleaned up. A finger monitor was attached.

The time in the intensive care unit was like some sort of stasis for me. Time there seemed to stretch into infinity. It was the exact opposite of Club Med. There was nothing friendly or warm or homelike about it. It was more like a submarine. And there we waited and waited and waited for some sign of improvement. I learned by watching the monitoring equipment what number indications were good and what were bad. Doctors I had never seen before appeared and disappeared like ghosts, over and over again, rarely the same doctor twice. It was so lonely without Dr. Laubenstein, without our home-health nurse. We sat and we waited. Joe couldn't speak too much because of the oxygen mask, and the wall unit made a great deal of noise. Every so often I would wander out to a waiting room for a break where there were ugly and uncomfortable plastic chairs. Occasionally there would be another person there, another care partner to a patient, but it looked like I was the only

AIDS care partner. Now and then I would come across someone weeping or just sitting and looking exhausted, and as I sat
there drinking putrid coffee from a machine, I wondered if I
looked as bad as they did.

Then there seemed to be a slight improvement. It was nothing dramatic. Joe's breathing seemed to ease somewhat. Blood
gasses were coming back a bit. It was decided that they would
take him from the unit and put him into a regular hospital room
a few floors down. I telephoned his mother and his sister, Laura,
to let them know the good news.

Just before Joe was moved from intensive care, an older
doctor I had never seen before asked me to come out to the
hallway. I thought we were going to begin battle over the
catheter once again. We stood in a part of the hospital by a
bank of elevators that was not as new as the rest, run-down
and unrestored. Naked fluorescent lights hung overhead and
cast a harsh light around us that seemed to suddenly end
within a few feet of us, giving way to dingy and dark corners.
A set of swinging doors were nearby that led into the intensive care unit, where Joe labored to breathe, and I was vague-
ly aware of the traffic in and out.

"Have the two of you ever had discussions about extraordinary means?" the doctor asked.

"Extraordinary means," I repeated, as if I had never heard the
words before or the doctor had just popped some very complicated medical phraseology on me. Then, I wanted to say, yes, yes,
we've laid awake at night holding hands talking about everything in the world. Why, do you know doctor, that he was able
to recite the poetry of T.S. Eliot to me in bed, holding my hand,

from memory? Doctor, do you know it was the most romantic and loving thing in the world to lie there in the dark with the spirit you love so much holding your hand while he recites poetry from memory? You should try it, doctor, there's nothing else like it in the world.

"Yes, certainly, we've discussed it. I am aware of his wishes. I have a power of attorney for health care."

"Did you ever discuss a respirator?"

I stood there in some degree of shock. I couldn't believe we were having this discussion. This is the discussion you imagine but never imagine really happening. I drew up these instruments for all my clients and now here I was, seeing what happened with them for the first time. Steve Bing, a dear friend and volunteer at GMHC had drawn ours up, but I never really thought about using them before. It was like hearing a death knell begin to ring in the distance, signaling to me that I would soon lose everything. It was like imagining a conversation with God. You could imagine having it, but when it actually happens, you are caught in awe, in a state of suspended disbelief.

"Yes, we discussed a respirator. He does not want to have it."

"You need to be sure," the doctor said.

"Well, what happens if we put him on the respirator? Can I take him off?

The doctor shook his head. "Once he is on, it would be difficult to remove it unless he could breathe on his own. If we put it on, it could be for 48 hours or it could be weeks; there's no way to tell."

The words hours or weeks echoed in my head. I thought of how much I loved Joe and how there was nothing I wouldn't do to have more time. More time. It wasn't fair. Everything I ever wanted in my life was in that intensive care room. Everything. I wanted more time. I would do anything for more time. Anything for a chance. He had been doing so well. I just wanted more time.

"No, no respirator," I said.

"Does he have parents?"

"They are not involved in this decision. He is not a minor. I am his power of attorney; I know his wishes. We've discussed this many times. He told me he never wants a respirator. He has signed a living will. We won't do a respirator."

The doctor, who I didn't know, walked away without saying anything else to me. The decision had come out and felt very natural. I had expected a fight from the doctor or from the hospital. I carried my legal documents with me at all times ready. In the end the decision I made was far easier legally, and far more difficult morally than I ever imagined either circumstance would be. I knew at the time that it was the right decision, and I knew how angry Joe would be with me if I had gone against his wishes. I also knew what a selfish gesture it would have been for me to place him on a respirator because I wanted more time. But I did so much want more time.

For years after that, during that vulnerable time before sleep comes at night, I would lie awake and wonder if I had done the right thing. What if I had put him on the respirator? Maybe in 48 hours he would have been taken off and would have had more time? What if they found a cure a year after I made the decision? What if I had put him on and we would have had two more years together? What if, what if, what if, what if, what if? There were endless scenarios to play out in my head again and again and again.

That night he suddenly deteriorated. By the time we got him to his new room, he was drenched in sweat, and there was a look of terror in his eyes, the kind anyone would get when they are breathing for all they are worth and getting no oxygen. Once safely hooked up, he entered a time that was neither deteriorating nor getting better. The doctor came in and examined him. He let me know that it was very, very serious and that Joe seemed to have some kind of infection of the lungs that was causing them to fill with fluid. Can't we give him a wide-spectrum antibiotic, I asked? I am sure the doctor wanted to say something sarcastic, like, Don't you think I've thought of that? But he quietly told me that one was being ordered. He then turned to the nurse and said, "If he wants morphine, give it to him. Give him anything he wants."

I knew then for certain that Joe was going to die. Doctors do this all the time. There are so many degrees to what we call euthanasia. Physician-assisted death does not only mean the kind that Dr. Kevorkian practices, but it is a good thing that his extreme example sets the stage for discussion. We are very cowardly as a society about discussing this, and though AIDS has brought discussion about it to the forefront, it is still not faced up to. Some doctors prescribe pills they know are being stockpiled for a final end. Other doctors let their patients know where they can get the information they will need to carry out a suicide with as little risk as possible. The brave physicians will order a plug pulled or withhold feeding from a tube. But some just are able to say, "Give him whatever he wants," and it will translate into a form of physician-assisted death, whether or not we want to talk about it.

As Joe's lungs began to fill with fluid, I called for that morphine whenever Joe wanted it, and they were very good about getting it to him. He would plateau for several hours and then suddenly get a little worse after a fit of bad breathing. I sat in a chair next to his bed, and we held hands all night. He kept trying to lower the metal guard at the side of the bed and asking me to lie down with him, but it was impossible with all the tubes. I frequently bathed his head. I did most of the talking because of the oxygen mask. We told each other several times that we loved each other. Sometimes he would take the oxygen mask off just to kiss me briefly.

In the morning it was raining a fine but constant mist. I had not bathed in about 40 hours, and I had been perspiring in buckets each time Joe took a turn for the worse or called out for morphine. I felt that I had to go home and bathe and feed our cats and then come back after a quick rest. Joe had not changed much in several hours. His GMHC buddy was coming to stay with him while I was gone. Before leaving, I asked him if there was anything he needed. "I'm just making a quick trip; you'll be OK?" He nodded. Appearing more animated than he had in hours, he lifted his oxygen mask and kissed me good-bye. I looked for The Look but didn't see it.

I took a cab home and immediately took a hot bath. I was fatigued. I wanted to lie down for a bit, but I was too restless and in some way too fatigued to rest. I was getting dressed to go back to the hospital. I stood looking in the mirror at my tired face and splashed on a few dollops of cologne to cover up my tiredness. When I put the bottle back on the shelf, I dropped it and it smashed into a million blue pieces on the floor just as the telephone began to ring.

Joe, his GMHC buddy said, was dead.

The time it took to take a simple bath was enough to make my entire life change. In a short hour and a half I had lost everything. It is remarkable how one's existence can change like that. How fragile one's consciousness really is, as if it were made up of nothing more than the substance of a snowflake, which under a microscope looks so powerfully crystalline and symmetrical—but with just a breath or a change in temperature is gone. Life is just a random sequence of events, and there are sublime moments where you are able to draw everything together just the way you want it and your universe has moved into place, and then in the next moment the universe continues to move, and it is all gone. The universe moves, oblivious to your state of happiness. And then you begin working on the next moment when you can again draw it all together. If you can.

The cab ride back to the hospital seemed to be occurring in slow motion and as I did it, I marveled that I could engage myself in all these mundane activities to be on my way to my dead spouse. I was, I think, in a bit of a state of shock. Every red light lasted an eternity. Every car in our way was an intolerable cruelty. I was so afraid they would take him away before I got there. A part of me really believed that if I got there soon enough, he wouldn't be dead after all.

I finally reached the hospital floor, and I felt everyone's eyes upon me as they watched me walk back to his room. It was with relief I found that they had left him there for me to come back to. For the first time in days there was no mask on his face, no hiss of oxygen. It was just clean and quiet. They let me be alone with him for a good while. I went into that room so quietly, but I was so angry with him for dying. And then looking at Joe, I was so surprised because he finally had The Look. It wasn't like he was really there at all. His body was there, but already it did not look like him. The absence of life is so unmistakable. The total void of any energy some-how makes the body smaller and so much more vulnerable. He was like some small sparrow, hit by a car and left at the side of the road. I held his hand as tightly and closely as I could, and I kept squeezing it as if I could pump the blood going again. I felt relief for him that his battle was over. At the same time I felt anger and rage that mine had just begun, and I had to fight the urge to yell at him. I didn't really un-derstand that he would just leave me like that. I couldn't be-lieve that he waited until I left the room. I blamed him. I let him know I loved him. Then slowly one of his eyes opened half way. I shut it and it opened again. I shut it again, and it stayed shut.

When I left the hospital I telephoned the funeral home and arranged for the body pickup. I went back to our apart-ment and telephoned his family. His mother said, "But I thought you said he was getting better." I told her that I had thought he was. I told her that Joe had directed that there would be no funeral and no memorial service. He said if I was up to it that I could have some sort of party if I wanted to. I never wanted to have a party. She asked if she should come out, and I replied that since there was no ceremony, there was no need. The body, I explained, was already on its way to being cremated. We hung up, and we never talked again. She told his family and her friends that Joe died of something other than AIDS. That was her failure as a mother to Joe; she could see how things affected only her. She never even bothered to ask me what I ended up doing with his body. I have kept his ashes, which are to be buried with my own.

That night I went home to several calls and the inevitable arrival of many flowers. My friend Bruce Anderson came and Tim Sweeney, though I didn't know what to say and I had nothing on hand to serve. My friends David Alvin and Rick Croll, one of the funniest and dearest men on earth, also came over and made my dinner and tucked me into bed before they left. It felt like I would make it through this if I could always have friends like them. They poured me a tall glass of gin before tucking me in. "I love you," I said to Rick. "I love you more," he said, because this is what we always said to each other since we had become friends.

After he and the others left I lay awake in an eerie apartment. Joe had never liked for the cats to sleep with us and had trained Rupert to stay away by squirting him with a plant sprayer when he came into the bedroom. Prior to our living together, both Ginger Pye and Rupert had always slept with me. Ginger Pye slept at my feet while Rupert slept like a lover in my arms, with his head tucked under my chin and a paw thrown across my chest in a gesture of possessive oblivion. Joe had always pretend-ed not to like the cats, but there was more than one day when I would come home to the apartment and find him asleep in bed with a cat on both sides of him, all three lost in slumber. Or where I would find the cat brush out and piles of hair in the waste can from a pleasant, long brushing.

"Rupert. Ru-u-u-pert," I called gently. Nothing happened. I waited. "Rupert. Time for bed Rupee." Still nothing. I kept up my calling, patiently waiting. Tears came into my eyes. Then I saw a movement by the door. The black-and-white form stood there silently looking at me. Slowly then Rupert walked to the foot of the bed and sat down. "Well, sure," his expression said, "he's dead. And now you want me back." I was grateful even if this did come with a lot of attitude. Then with a quick leap, he jumped on the foot of the bed, walked up the length of my body, lay down and put his head under my chin. He began to purr while I began to cry.

Joseph and Amy Sloan had become close after meeting at the People With AIDS Conference in San Francisco, but they never saw each other again. Amy died in November 1986. They were reunited in an August 1987 issue of *Newsweek* magazine, called the "Faces of AIDS." Amy's photograph was on the cover; Joseph's was inside.

The day after Joseph died, I had him cremated. I picked up the ashes the day after that. They were much heavier than I ex-pected them to be. I took the photograph Janet Beller had shot and had a frame made for it. It cost a fortune, and I thought that if Joe were still alive, he would have killed me for spending the last money we had on a frame.

I got a note from Janet Beller that stood out among all the others. It read:

Dear Mark,

The day we met I was so touched by both you and Joseph and by the compassion I felt existed between you that I actually felt compelled to do that portrait.

After it was delivered I became nervous that perhaps I'd made a mistake in sending Joseph a portrait of himself so thin and ill.

I cried when I got your note, but was relieved to hear that you both were pleased to have the portrait. It is a keepsake of Joseph and one that shows the kind of stuff life is worth living for.

I will remember you both.

Janet

The day after I collected Joe, I went away. When I came back a week later I realized what a mistake it was to have left all the flowers people sent. They had all withered and died, and there was something like Charles Dickens's Miss Havisham about the place. It was like a flower morgue. I tossed them all away realizing I'd made my first of what would be many mistakes on the road to wellness. I cleaned them all out, feeling terrible the whole time. I'd had my time away. I finished and sat down on the couch, where we had spent every evening when I first came home, where I could tell him the troubles of my day, and I wondered, *Now what?*

Since then I often think back to that night in 1978 when I saw him in that damned bar down in the Village and I tried so hard to get his attention and he didn't see me. It had been as if I were in another dimension. I still wonder now that he is gone if the shoe isn't on the other foot and he is there somewhere nearby and is trying to get my attention, but I'm just unable see him. I like that sort of symmetry.

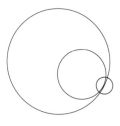

P A R T    T H R E E

D O I N G    T H E
R I G H T    T H I N G S

*"O mother, mother make my bed,*
*O make it soft and narrow;*
*My love has died for me today*
*I'll die for him tomorrow. "*

~BARBARA ALLEN'S CRUELTY ANONYMOUS~

## THE QUILT

Joe died in June 1987. In November of that year the AIDS memorial quilt would be on display on the Mall in front of the White House for the first time as part of a national gay and lesbian march on Washington. In my mind a quilt was something that belonged on a bed, but the idea that it would be a memorial to people who had died of AIDS struck me as quaint. I've never been big on "process," and the quilt clearly was an institutionalized effort at processing everyone's grief. I didn't make fun of it; I just didn't take it seriously. I also worried about the kind of symbolism it might represent to people with HIV who were living. "I don't want to end up with my name on that quilt," said Vito Russo, a friend I'd made just after Joe died.

For anyone connected with AIDS, however, a meeting with the Quilt is an inevitability. In the six months since Joe died, I had not stopped thinking of him for any period of any day, and my mourning hung around me like a heavy perfume. So when my friend Bruce Anderson called to say he had arranged for us to meet down in Washington and attend the march, it seemed like a good idea. I went to Washington with an open mind but did not think that the simple and sweet notion stirred up in San Francisco would in any way move me. I met up with Bruce and Tim Sweeney, who would soon become the executive director of GMHC. As I marched to the Mall Joe sat at the edge of my consciousness as I silently communicated with him from time to time imagining what he would have said about this or that. It was a great comfort thinking of him walking next to me. In front of the White House I ran into Todd. Our relationship had lasted less than a year and ended in 1982, and I hadn't seen him since. We chatted only briefly, though I couldn't concentrate because my eyes were scanning his entire body, looking for any signs that he might be sick. It was a hot day, and he was wearing a tank top. I was pleased that it looked like he had gained weight, and since he was showing so much skin, I saw no KS lesions. He had always been an example of the Peter Pan syndrome, a little boy who wasn't going to grow up, which can be charming. At some age, though, the Peter Pan motif begins looking a little tattered. But ironically now, if anything, Todd seemed even more boyish than he had five years earlier. In the few minutes that it took us to say hello and have some awkward conversation, I surmised that his attitude reminded me a bit of my boyhood friend, Neil, who had just found out that he was HIV-positive. Of course, I couldn't ask if he were HIV-positive; it would have been too obvious that I was feeling threatened. It would also be obvious I hadn't tested. So we just exchanged pleasantries and went on our way, and I walked away trying to reassure myself that he really, really looked OK.

Tim Sweeney and I decided to go to see the quilt display together, the idea of which began to intimidate me just a bit. I had heard that people were there to hand out tissues to those who could not control their emotions and the idea of this made me uneasy. I wasn't all that comfortable with my own grief, much less seeing others display theirs. I had stopped going to memorials or funeral services entirely. But when we got to the expanse of lawn around the Washington Monument, the sight of the quilt laid out for so far, each panel the size of a grave, was nothing less than awe-inspiring.

All my earlier notions about the value of the quilt melted away under that Washington autumn sun. Each panel seemed to tell a story that was compelling. A cowboy shirt sewn onto one, a rainbow on another, a baby blanket and rattle on another, and on and on and on, seemingly acres of lives and stories and the grief that surrounded their sad conclusion seen in the nervous people walking around the edges of each set of panels. Each panel had so many lives attached to it, I thought. A mother, a father, a sister, a brother, a lover, a friend, a son, a daughter—they were all out there carrying with them the memory of the person in this panel and that panel and the next panel. For each panel, I thought, there must be at least five other lives that were rocked by this death. All of that pain. Surely, I reasoned, if the epidemic kept up, there would be no end to the blanket of pain and loss spreading across America.

There was the kind of hush on the Mall that is usually experienced in a cathedral. It is the same kind of hush one becomes aware of at a cemetery or at the Vietnam War memorial, which is similar but different. Because standing in the middle of the display could almost swallow you up, and you wonder what names are there that you know and what names you know are yet to come. If your heart is beating, it cannot help but to be touched by all the personal effects attached to the panels, all the love that went into each one.

Timbo and I had said nothing to one another upon entering the walkways among the panels, but at one point he did come up from behind and put his arms around me, and we had a good cry. I cried for Joe and for all the people represented by the panels and for all those yet to come, and I was glad someone had given someone the charge of carrying a box of Kleenex to those of us in need. There were tears for myself too. Looking around, I had to wonder if I had HIV and had to wonder who would be making a quilt panel for me and when? Unlike the Vietnam War memorial, except for the men still missing in action, the war is over and the memorial static. For us, it just goes on and on with no end in sight. How many acres will need to be covered?

At the other end of the mall, there were the inevitable stage and speakers set up. I was never attracted to listening to soapbox speakers expound endless theories of government corruption or conspiracy. But the speakers talked about the unity of our experience and the depth of our feelings and everyone was profoundly moved. We were told that this was the last time the quilt would be assembled in its entirety—that it had become too big and too heavy to be ever reunited again in one spot—a metaphor for the epidemic itself. It had just become too big and too heavy to be viewed from any one spot. You could never get an understanding of it in its entirety.

I went back to New York feeling as if I had been born again. Nothing was ever the same for me after that weekend. It was a smart thing that someone did to bring us all together for that weekend and have us see the quilt in its entirety because it gave those of us who were there a sense of identity about our gay selves and what was happening to us. It also made it clear once and for all that a new subculture was emerging, one that was not built around being gay but about experiencing HIV. Once home I was like a Jehovah's Witness, anxious to talk to people about what the weekend had meant and what the beauty of the quilt was like there on the Mall in Washington. I telephoned my friend Mark but instead got his boyfriend, David. Desperate to talk about it, I launched into a lengthy description of my weekend—the quilt panels, the speakers, the camaraderie of hundreds of thousands of feet marching together because they knew each other's pain, the sheer feeling of power connected with so many thousands of people who, through their own experience, knew how you felt.

"Well," he sighed, "we were going to go, but we just got back from Spain, and we were so-o-o tired. So we just stayed home and had sex, and that was our contribution to gay rights."

I was so stunned, I didn't know what to say. This wasn't about gay rights. David's utter failure to "get it" just pushed me over the edge. It was insulting, not just to me, but to every quilt panel I had seen.

"Just have Mark call me," I said. I hung up, and I never spoke to David again.

While on display in Washington in 1987, the quilt had many thousands of panels, each one 3 feet by 6 feet, the size of a grave. When laid out, it covered several football fields. While strolling along the walkways, one had a clear view of the White House, and one had to assume the White House had a clear view of us. But in that fall of 1987 no one from the White House came out to see the quilt. In fact, the quilt was displayed again on the Mall during the Bush administration years, but again no one came from the White House. Finally in 1996, when once again displayed in its entirety on the Mall, President Bill Clinton, first lady Hillary Rodham Clinton, Vice President Al Gore, and Tipper Gore did come to see the quilt. The first lady, the vice president, and Mrs. Gore all read names. For all the jokes that parodied the president's statement to anguished voters that "he feels their pain," unlike his predecessors, he at least signaled us that he indeed did. It should be noted that during the 1992 Republican National Convention, Barbara Bush wore a red ribbon while seated in the audience, but when she went to the podium and the television cameras were trained on her in anticipation of giving her speech, she removed it. I wish it were as easy for the rest of us.

## MEET YOUR LEARNING CURVE

Getting over the death of someone who is important is not an event; it's a process. But our culture is geared to immediate gratification in so many ways, and grieving is no different. I think a part of me believed that if I did all the "right things" I would be OK. People who were grief-struck were just people who could not cultivate the art of doing the "right things," but I was absolutely confident that I could do this.

The day after Joe died I had all the medical equipment and paraphernalia taken away that same day. The day after that I went and picked up the ashes, took them home, not sure what I would do with them since his only response to my queries in this regard were that I should do what I wanted to with them, and I wasn't sure what that was. Maybe I should scatter them in the ocean, I thought. Or maybe have them interred somewhere he would have liked. Well, I figured, I had time on my side. It's not like they had an appointment to be somewhere. I would put that decision off until later. Besides, I knew really that I couldn't give them up. I knew that they had to be buried with my own ashes at some point. I just didn't know where that point might be.

I rearranged all the furniture, doing away with all the decisions that *we* made, and putting furniture where *I* thought it needed to be. In fact, there is a very painful adjustment that takes a great deal of time and effort, saying "I" instead of "we." Your identity undergoes an unwelcome transformation.

I listened to my instincts and told myself that I should get away. The day after I collected his ashes, I went to stay with Doris Taussig, a 75-year-old friend of ours in the Pines on Fire Island. Doris was a longtime volunteer at GMHC on the hotline, which is how she met both of us. After she heard what happened she invited me to go out there and spend a few days. While I was there she told me that when Joe and I were first thinking of dating, he called her and asked her if he could come and stay with her for a weekend. He said that he needed to decide whether it was the right thing to do—dating a man who wasn't sick, dating at all while he was so sick. Thankfully, during his visit, Doris put her two cents worth in and she told him that she thought it was a lucky thing to find love and that one shouldn't question the circumstances too severely, and then Joe came back to New York, and we began our relationship. I hadn't known about this until she told me. It was like finding a gift, hidden for me by Joe until after he died. She told me while we were dressed for dinner, sitting in her living room having a gin and tonic. So there I was, three days after cremating his body, staying in the same guesthouse in the same room in the same bed but now trying to decide how to end our relationship. Accident and Providence can really be amazingly symmetrical.

Doris recalls that I was a bit crazed. I remember walking walking and walking. I would walk on the beach back and forth, up and down, until the sun came up, and then I would sleep a few hours and begin walking all over again. Fire Island being a very narrow but very long island that allows you a lot of walking space. There are no cars, and there are deer who will walk right up to you if they think you have anything to eat. The beach was long then, though today it is more abbreviated by storms. I would lay my footprints down and then sit and watch them be washed over by the tide, and then I would lay them down again, as if I could prove something about mortality by this exercise. One of the nights I met a man on the beach—a very handsome black man near my own age. We didn't really say anything, but he kissed me and I kissed him back. I wanted to be held by someone else; I wanted for all my pain to be behind me, and most of all, in the middle of it I wanted to know what I was doing just a few days after the death of my lover kissing another man. I just wanted to forget. I just wanted to remember.

When I left Fire Island, I treated myself to a trip back on the sea plane, which picked me up on the beach and flew me back to Manhattan. I charged it on a credit card that had just enough space left on it for the extravagance. I was going to pay for it with money I would get from a speaking engagement I had the next day. My sea plane landed in the East River just within sight of Club Med, where we had spent our last few moments together. I took a cab to our apartment, which was eerily quiet. I grabbed a suit in a flash, went back down to the cab which was waiting for me, and then to the airport for a flight to Boston. That felt very jet-setty. The next day I gave my speech, the fee for which paid for the sea plane and the week on Fire Island. I told myself that this had all been healthy and had all been part of the set of magical "right things to do."

But peace wasn't coming all that easily, and those months after Joe died would have a sort of unreal cast to them. Every day when I woke up, I would have to go through a mental exercise to tell me what had happened so that the day seemed real. You wake up alone and say to yourself, "I'm alone because Joe got sick, he went into the hospital, he died, and he's not coming back." And you had to say this to yourself every day, sometimes more than once a day. That was a pretty big dose of reality to start the day. Then I would lie there a bit and let it sink in. A cat or two would wander into bed and begin purring and nuzzling and as wonderful as this is, it becomes painfully apparent that the little ball of fur is no match for waking up with someone you love.

The house is much quieter than you remember it being. You open your eyes in the morning and are surprised at how cold the bed is with only you there. Early morning was always a special time for us. We didn't make love when we went to bed at night too often. But we would always wake up around 5 A.M. and wordlessly find each other for a fervent and quiet communion. We'd fall back to sleep until the other morning would begin.

But now by myself, I would begin a morning routine that definitely involved turning on a radio or television just for the sound of another person. You begin to adjust to this new life as if you've just gone into some kind of institutional living and you are still getting used to where things are. You keep coming across clothing that isn't yours, books, and personal effects, and remind yourself that you have to do something about that soon, knowing that you are putting it off only because it is the beginning of a long process of healing that you'd rather not admit you have to go through.

Memory has a dual nature when it comes to the loss of a loved one. The mind works to remember the things you want to remember—the smell of hair, the touch of skin, the sound of a voice, while at the same time working to relieve itself of the bad. Unfortunately, after a loss, even the things you want to remember cause pain, and your loneliness takes on the character of "white noise"—a noise that is there but isn't. And each dwelling on a memory causes this noise to echo in your head, until a crescendo is reached, reminding you that you are alone, that you have lost someone forever. He or she may be your son or your daughter, your mother or your father, your brother or your sister, or as in my case, your lover. It is that touch you hold so special, the voice next to your ear in the middle of the night, the eyes that speak to you without saying a word. It was good-bye to the most special love I have known—saying good-bye to the poetry in my night. There are definitely times in the wake of a loss when you wonder if you want to go on living at all. It is a natural part of loss.

One day back in 1984, as had become my custom, I was walking home from my job at the investment firm. I took a route through the park, gaining entrance at Fifth Avenue and 59th Streets near the Plaza Hotel and walking in a diagonal to exit at 72nd Street and Central Park West. From there it was a short walk to my home at 75th Street. It was a pleasant and healthy walk, and I did it in all sorts of inclimate weather. On this particular winter day, I was walking at around 6 P.M., and it was dusk. There was a dull orange sun setting, and the rest of the sky was a tepid gray. The park was particularly deserted and I strolled along, daydreaming about whatever it is I dreamed about while walking across the Park, usually about how much I disliked my boss. Near the top of a hill close to 72nd Street in the middle of the Park, I was walking and gazing at the ground when suddenly I became aware of someone standing in front of me and looked up to see three kids standing about six feet away from me, no older than 18 years old, standing in a semicircle, blocking my pathway. I stopped and we looked at one another. They said nothing, but in the fading sun I could clearly see the reflection of their knife blades. They were each looking at me and held up the knives and smiled.

Well, there was nothing I could do that could match up to that gesture. I had once heard that muggers are sometimes frightened away if you start talking crazy to yourself, but amazingly, I could think of nothing crazy to say. I didn't look too tough. Wearing a trench coat, loafers, a gray double-breasted suit with a red-and-gray bow tie and tortoise-shell glasses, I looked exactly like the other 99,999 27-year-old lawyers in New York. I didn't know what to do or how to respond. If they had been nine feet away, I would have just tossed out my wallet. If they had been three feet away, I would have screamed. But six feet away just caught me dumb, and I stopped and stared at them. My eyes met the eyes of the boy in the center, and as they did, I had the very strong sense that he wasn't going to kill me. I did not lock my gaze with his; it was only a quick and tidy assessment. And then I moved forward and stepped between he and his neighbor and kept on walking. As I walked, I overcame the almost irresistible impulse to look over my shoulder. I walked down the path, wondering what it would feel like to have a knife blade at my throat and someone pull it. I wondered if I would feel anything. I wondered if I was about to find out.

Reaching the bottom of the hill, I stopped walking. I hadn't heard any footsteps in back of me. I finally turned around and saw only the brown winter grass, the gray sky, and the last filaments of the orange sunset.

"Jesus," I said, a rare exclamation from me. I turned and walked brusquely toward Tavern on the Green, thanking God that someone had had the foresight to put a bar in the park. What a good idea.

I think now of the AIDS epidemic a lot like that day. There I was, walking around, looking at the ground, minding my own business, indistinguishable from anyone else. I had the same worries, the same fears, the same things made me happy and sad. But all of a sudden there was a wall of confrontation, one I had never imagined and for which I had no plan. I acted only on instinct, stupid or not. It is not a heroic reaction, just lucky. It was after all only a matter of chance that I did not become a New York homicide statistic that day. It is likewise a matter of chance that I haven't died of AIDS. Nothing I did fended them off unless in fact they were intimidated by my bow tie. Maybe they saw someone else and ran off. I'll never know.

The epidemic has not been scared off, but so far it has kept its hands off me. I still walk down that long hill. But unlike that day, I take the opportunity as I have in these pages to peek over my shoulder. What I see is difficult. But there is no question, pain or not, I've decided I definitely want to go on living.

One month to the day after Joe died, I went to stay for the July 4 weekend with close friends John Bennett and Linda Coleman in Southampton.

My first night there I had my first dream about Joe. I was in a room full of young men, and the atmosphere was one of a subdued cocktail party. I didn't seem to know anyone, and I sauntered through the crowd with a drink in hand, looking for an inviting or familiar face. For reasons that escape me, everyone was wearing a crew neck sweater, though each one was a different shade. Then, as I was looking around, the men in front of me moved and through the crowd, wearing the maroon crew neck sweater my mother had bought him, was Joe.

He looked great. He was smiling already when our eyes met. Upon his seeing me, his expression did not change much, and though I could tell he was glad to see me, he did not have my obvious feeling of surprise and delight. I walked over to him and said hi, sheepishly, as if I had just run into him after a brief break up of our relationship. He replied hi back, and then we both stared at the ground and shuffled our feet back and forth while a heavy silence hung around us. It was one of those situations where there was so much to say, it was difficult and awkward to begin by saying anything. I wanted to touch him so badly, but I was afraid to.

"It is so nice to see you again." I said.

"It's nice to see you too."

A handsome blond man in a light green sweater was hanging

close by. I put my hand on Joe's arm and moved him closer to me so that the blond couldn't eavesdrop.

"Look," I said, "I know we talked about it and planned for it, but it has been nothing like the way we anticipated it. It has been so tough, Joe. You have no idea what I've been through the last month. It has been so much harder than either one of us imagined it would be."

"I know it has," he said. These words comforted me a great deal, because I could tell by the clarity of his expression that he really did know everything I had gone through and that he was full of empathy. Then he said something that perplexed me. "It has been tough on me too."

I was embarrassed. Here he clearly knew what I had been through, and yet I had no idea what his ordeal had been like. I could not give him the same empathy he gave me, and I knew that it showed. Of course, I thought, being dead, he gets to know what's going on with me all the time. How could I know what it has been like for him?

"Well, listen," I said, taking his arm again and steering him away, "maybe now that we've seen each other like this and talked—maybe we could get back together. I would like that so much, Joe. Maybe we could just start seeing each other again."

He stopped walking with me and gently took his arm away. "I can't," he said. "I'm with someone else now." And then he pointed to the handsome blond in the green sweater. Joe left me and walked over to the other man, and they both turned to me and smiled. I woke up—not very happy.

That sort of sums up 1987. It was a year of confusion for me

about what the hell exactly had happened. I don't think I understood what happened to Joe. I'm still not sure I understand
it. He was just gone. One day there, the next day not. And the
right things were becoming less clear. I put all his pictures away,
then, lonely for him, I brought them all back out again. This
went back and forth for months. Sometimes I would wear his
clothes to feel close to him, and other times I would put them
all away as if I were going to rid myself of them. It was a con-
fusing time. The rest of 1987 was like that: a steep learning curve.

*35,818 new cases of AIDS were diagnosed*
*21,074 more people died*
*A cumulative total of 106,994 cases were diagnosed*
*62,101 people were dead of AIDS in America*

## ANOTHER LESSON IN THE PARK

New Yorkers really need Central Park. I was no different. As I said, after Joe died I was sure that I was doing all the right things. I took a little trip. I kept busy, and I had been a good student with my learning curve. My decisions were all clear-cut. But clearly, feeling no better, I had screwed up somewhere and the thought of this created a growing problem. My big mistake here was that I didn't realize how very, very angry I was.

At a time like this everyone is full of advice. It is well intended but rarely serves to do anything but confuse. The range of prescriptions by well-wishers was often difficult to hear, and more often contradictory. People encourage you to either make big changes or not to change much at all because you may regret it later on, not being yourself and all. When Joe was alive we often toyed with the idea of moving to California. It was a practical impossibility given the fact that I didn't have any job prospects there, we had no car, and most of all we had no money but lots of debt. There had been months where we lived off credit cards. Still, it had been a fun fantasy, particularly in months of rain, sleet, and snow that New York serves up without apology from Christmas until tax time. Now that he was gone, I carried on that fantasy myself and thought moving might not be a bad idea. My job was so oppressive to me that I found myself doing it with less dedication than before. GMHC was growing by leaps and bounds, and I now had a staff of five and a few hundred volunteers. It was difficult to keep my mind on the mundane machinations that come with growing bureaucracy. It was still a caring environment, but there were now several people working in at least three different sites and the feeling of familial support that had been there when Barry Davidson and the others all met in the kitchen for coffee was diluted. And I needed support. Certainly, deathbed wills became exceedingly difficult and depressing, as if they weren't in the first place. Sometimes I found myself angry that the client had gotten himself sick in the first place, a notion only one step away from the anger I was really feeling—anger with Joe for getting sick and for dying and of course for leaving me.

That anger began to catch up with me at odd moments, and mostly on weekends when I had to face life alone in my apartment and was mostly turned inward. Although I had done everything "right" after he died—all the "healthy" things—I still found that I would come home from work and sit on the couch in my work clothes until it was dark. Coming home from work was a hard time. When Joe was alive I ran home so I could get there sooner. When he died I tried not to come home until late. Because Joe would always be waiting for me when I came home from work and now he wouldn't. He'd wait for me while sitting on the couch. If I was five minutes late, he'd ask why, because regular timing is very important to people who are mainly homebound. He'd put his hand on the couch when I came through the door and say, "Come and sit here and let me hold you." And he'd actually be eager to hear about every detail of my day. I would mix a drink for me and a health shake for him, and we'd put some saxophony-jazzy thing on the stereo. So coming home without that was always hard, especially by Friday night. Without turning on the lights, I would go to the freezer and re- turn to the couch and eat an entire container of Häagen-Dazs ice cream in the dark. The stereo remained quiet, and dinner seemed irrelevant.

But one night it was not a matter of anger turned inward. I had been to the home of some friends for dinner and had had too much to drink, which I did a lot of back then. New York is such an easy place to drink too much because you don't have to drive you just have to look cogent on the subway, which given the competition is not so very hard. It was late and after dinner I stopped at a bar, an arena in which I had never been success- ful in my socialization efforts. It only served to depress me fur- ther and make me feel more lonely than I had been before. In my head I told Joe off for being so selfish as to get sick. I hated myself for being so sad and lonely. I went home but I was so restless and angry, I couldn't be there. I couldn't just sit there in the quiet dark. I didn't want to stay there. I hated it. I was mad at everyone and everything. I left the apartment with a barely controlled rage and began walking all over the upper west side. It grew late, and I was near the park. I looked at it, so dark and foreboding at night when it's so inviting and pleasant during the day. I looked at my watch and saw that it was 1:30 A.M. I walked across Central Park West and into the dark void.

I don't know what I expected to find. I mean, I figure if three guys can pull knives on me in broad daylight, there would certainly be trouble waiting for me at night. And I wanted that trouble. I felt sorry for anyone who wanted to mess with me. I knew that the kind of trouble people usually met with in a dark park in the middle of the night was not good for them, but I didn't care. I didn't give a shit if I got hurt, but I really wanted to fight someone. I walked for an hour in the park and never saw another person. I finally was exhausted and walked home and fell asleep. In the morning when I woke up, I realized that I had better move my ass to California. Change could only be good.

## JEWISH DOCTOR

"Hello, Mr. Senak?"

"Yes."

"This is Mrs. so-and-so down in Memphis?" She spoke this in that uniquely Southern manner, where almost every sentence carries the inflection of a question rather than a statement.

"Yes."

"Mr. Senak, I got you listed as a speaker tomorrow at the Peabody Hotel on AIDS, and there are these initials here behind your name, and I don't know what they mean?"

"What initials are those?" I asked, genuinely perplexed.

"JD" she said.

"Oh," I said. I often forgot the fact that I was a lawyer. Even though it had been a few years since I passed the bar exam in the state of New York, it still seemed like a foreign title to me. "That stands for juris doctor."

"What?" she sounded genuinely perplexed.

"Juris doctor."

"Jewish doctor?" she asked with some amazement.

"No," I said, "but you just made my mother the happiest woman in America."

"What?"

"No," I repeated, "JD stands for juris doctor. It's a law degree."

"Oh, I see. I'm sorry," she said.

"That's OK," I said.

This conversation occurred on the eve of my move to California in May 1988. President Ronald Reagan had only just given his first talk about AIDS, despite the fact that there were 30,000 diagnosed Americans. The response of the United States government had been maddeningly slow, especially when you compared it with the response to Legionnaires' disease a decade earlier. It was expected in a way, yet still we were a community incredulous that we were actually being treated as badly as we thought we were going to be. It made a lot of us quite angry; some more than others. In 1987 ACT UP was formed, with activists getting arrested, being where they weren't supposed to be, in everyone's face as much as possible, tossing blood on the carpets of Congress people and government bureaucrats. Thank God.

The move to the West Coast was taking me away from all that, however. The chaos of moving across the country was too all-consuming for me to be very distracted by the current round of injustices or stupidity or arrogant ignorance expressed by members of government. The logistics of packing, finding a place in L.A., and the cost of the whole thing was all completely absorbing. That was why I took the speaking engagement for the National Institute of Allergy and Infectious Diseases and with anyone else who asked me and offered me money. I needed money for the move. While the idea took root right after he died, as the year went on. I thought more and more about moving to Southern California. I had visited my friends Mike Lombardo and Allen Wallace once while Joe was sick. Mike had worked with me for a while at the firm where I met Jeff, my first AIDS death. For a while when I was in law school and still a floating secretary at the law firm, I had been Mike's secretary. After we both left the firm in 1981 he went to Home Box Office in New York, and we became best friends. Then in 1987 Mike was transferred by HBO to L.A., and Allen, his lover, followed several months later. It had ripped my heart out when Mike got transferred because I knew he wouldn't be in New York when Joe died and I would most need his support. But now I looked at it as if Mike had blazed a trail for me to show me the way out of my unhappiness. Allen Wallace was the nice young man who opened the door to me at Richard's apartment four years before and to so many nightmares afterward.

Los Angeles had seduced me, like any good lover, when I was pretty vulnerable. A few weeks after Joe died, as part of the right-things regimen, I went and stayed again with Mike and Allen at their home in Laurel Canyon. The weather was spectacular, and there was an exhilarating sense of liberation connected with having a big old American car that would move fast when I pressed the pedal. It was a far cry from the stoic passivity offered by the New York subway or the Long Island Railroad.

There was charm in everything about L.A. We'd wake up in the morning and have coffee together, which I often made because, being on New York time, I was up the earliest. We would read the paper. Allen would make me a beautiful breakfast. I don't mean beautiful in the sense that it was delicious, though it was; I mean beautiful in that it was aesthetically pleasing. One morning he made me an omelet and a hibiscus sitting off to the side, like it had grown there naturally. It was the kind of thoughtfulness that was so unique to Allen. It is a rare man that thinks of such a touch and who knows his audience so well that he knows that the gesture will be enormously appreciated. It is one of the things I loved so much about Allen. He could speak to your heart that way, just the way he did when he opened the door to Richard's apartment that day. Then too his actions were filled with nuance that communicated a desire to make everyone comfortable in hidden and subtle ways.

By contrast, my breakfasts in New York did not often begin with a hibiscus flower on my plate. But in L.A., Allen made it seem commonplace. Here is your breakfast and your flower. After breakfast I'd nurse a coffee alone on the back deck until everyone was gone to work while I finished every morsel of the morning paper, a luxury offered by vacation time that is never truly attainable the rest of the year. Everything about it was such an antithesis to my life in New York. Hummingbirds gathered on the back deck to poke their long noses into the reddest flowers they could find, of which there were many. Birds made their presence known through a lot of song, sometimes frankly too much. In New York, well, you could hear sirens and garbage trucks and subway rumblings underneath the street, all of which were admittedly very comforting sounds to me but not like these were. Even the newspaper was different. At the bottom of the newspaper column in *The New York Times,* it reads "Continued on page 6" but in the *Los Angeles Times,* it always says "*Please* turn to page 6" (emphasis my own). This subtlety was not lost on me. New York had reached a point, I decided, where it took more energy from me than it gave me. L.A., however, even in its newspaper, seemed to want to be restorative.

Besides, I rationalized, I didn't think I could take one more New York dreary February. February in New York was the worst, sitting on a heated subway seat in a winter coat like a baked potato wrapped in tin foil on a grill, only to go upstairs to a more than bracing wind fleecing your clothes like they were gauze and facing a street corner that was a sea of slush longing to leak into your shoes the first chance it had. L.A. was so nice in February. On Santa Monica Boulevard in West Hollywood you can face east and see the mountains in the distance covered by snow. As the late afternoon draws to a close, the snow captures the pink of the setting sun and glows a healthy Los Angeleno countenance. Later I would come to miss all those horrible things about New York in desperate fashion, and I would have to come to admit that the only three things I liked about L.A. were the climate, the climate, and the climate. But then, I was being seduced, and as in any seduction, it seemed like the right thing to do at the time. So I was going to move to this glorious mecca of hummingbirds and tanned bodies, where no buildings held memories of deathbed wills.

But there was one serious impediment to the move. I didn't know if I was infected or not. I lived countless nights lying in bed thinking about Joe and actually wanting to join him "on the other side" but afraid of the road I would have to take to get there. I did not want to be sick, but I had no idea whether lurking somewhere in my bloodstream, there was a small and insidious virus eating away at my immune system until one day I would develop that long-anticipated persistent cough that would swell into pneumocystis pneumonia. Or the inevitable mark would suddenly appear on an ankle, an arm, or between my toes, and it would be biopsied and turn out of course to be Kaposi's sarcoma. I lay awake at night thinking about it, wondering what was going on inside my body, whether one day it would betray me and how. Wondering whether something from my past would come back to haunt me. Wondering why I was left and others were gone. Wondering if there would be anyone to take care of me if and when I got sick. These were days and nights of uncertainty.

At least Mike and Allen would be there. When I moved to New York at 21, I had known only one woman from my German class. This time I would know at least two people. I began buying the *Los Angeles Times* (Please turn to page 6) and combing it for job opportunities. Within six months I found a position at St. Mary Medical Center in Long Beach to administer an outpatient HIV program. I interviewed by telephone and was offered the job but came out to make sure I would like it. I called my New York friends from L.A. to tell them that the deal was on, that I was moving in one month to Los Angeles. Despite the fact that I had talked about this for months, everyone seemed truly shocked. The truth was so was I.

There was no better person to drive cross country with me than Rick Croll. It seemed as if we were good friends from the first day we had ever laid eyes on each other at GMHC. We always laughed a lot when we were together, even if we were only rehashing old movie lines from *All About Eve* or *The Women* or *I Love Lucy* episodes. We had a theory that there was no situation in life for which Lucy and Ethel had not already prepared you, and on this point we were authorities. Who better then to ask to make the drive with me on my trip to Los Angeles? When I asked him, he didn't even hesitate to say yes, telling me that he had never been west of Pennsylvania.

But there was an intervening complication. Between the time that Rick tucked me into my bed the night that Joe died and the time of my move 11 months later, he had been diagnosed with AIDS. I hadn't even known that he was infected with HIV. People didn't talk about it as easily then as they do today. "Are you positive or negative?" a date will ask. "About what?" I like to say. But back then, it was still considered an issue of privacy and you just didn't come out and ask. And people like me didn't ask because we hadn't been tested and didn't want anyone talking us into it. If the subject came up, I avoided it. I was more afraid of taking a test than I was of waking up and finding a purple lesion on my body.

Rick had been sick but not seriously ill. He was using aerosol pentamadine as a prophylaxis against getting another bout of pneumonia. Today most people take a pill as a prophylaxis, but the new fad that had hit in 1987 was an antibiotic that had to be breathed in through a handheld vaporizer. Joe had used this method. The problem was that it had to be monitored by a nurse because a person's blood pressure could suddenly rise and cause complications. Nothing comes without its side effects. Since we thought that it would take us a week on the road and then another week of Rick visiting, Rick would have to find some way to take his treatment on the road. But he discussed it with his doctor and decided that missing a treatment wouldn't be fatal. But that was the way people with AIDS had to be about their lives. You had to be very careful about the plans you made.

I was getting kind of manicky right before leaving. I would pack a box halfway and then start to pack another. I started out organized, labeling everything, but melted down the closer the time came to actually leaving. I was scared to death. I was very conscious that I was leaving behind all but two of the people who loved me and who would take care of me should anything happen. If I got diagnosed in California, what would happen to me? I knew only Mike and Allen, and I couldn't stand the thought of becoming a burden to them. Two people could not take the place of two dozen who would go to the mat for me in New York. What if I piled all my shit into a truck and moved to L.A. and got sick a month later? My childhood friend Neil would be only 500 miles away, but he had called with the news that he was sick now too. In all likelihood I would be taking care of him, not vice versa. And too I would be completely out of money. I had cashed in my hard-won retirement account and borrowed $1,000 from my friend K.C. McDaniel, and that was all the money I had in the world. It would be gone by the time I arrived in Los Angeles. As it was, I needed to start my new job within a few days of arriving just to make sure I could still eat. But as much as this frightened me I again found it repugnant to give into the idea that this virus was going to control my life to such an extent that I couldn't make normal life decisions just like everyone else. If I wanted to move to the West Coast, then, damn it, I was going to move.

*The New York Times* ran a little good-bye piece about me in their regular column about attorneys called "At the Bar." David Margolick interviewed me at length and wrote a very kind and thoughtful piece about my "retirement" from AIDS work. They sent a photographer on a day when I was packing. I was nervous and hungover. From that they drew a pen and ink drawing of me to run with the column, showing me looking ten years older than I was and with a forehead so big, you could get 125 channels on it if you used it for a satellite dish. The piece, however, was very touching, and David Margolick really captured what I had meant to express while we talked. Looking back on the work that had been done by me and my colleagues, I had to stop and marvel. We were people who cared so much about the injustice of what was happening that we overcame our fears and took care of each other when no one else was going to do it.

We had opened disease-specific organizations and kept them open and given them money to help people before society even knew there was a problem. We overcame stigma and ignorance and discrimination, and I said then what I say now: I believe when people get in touch with the part of themselves that God put there, they can make miracles happen. And every day that we kept the doors open and gave people help, we made miracles happen. The piece came out a few weeks before I left, and it was a wonderful send-off. Today in my mind those sentiments are only more confirmed amid the cynical attitudes of people in the community about HIV services and the people who deliver them. It seems we are caught between the arts of creation and destruction when it comes to these community-based organizations. We created them because the mainstream was letting us down. They did great things and had to grow with the epidemic to serve all the people in need. When they became big and were no longer warm and fuzzy little grassroots organizations, they fell prey to avalanches of criticism from the community from which they sprang. Some of the criticism deserved, a good deal of it nothing more than the byproduct of a weird HIV contest at times—a product of the "My Pain Is Bigger Than Your Pain" syndrome. AIDS gave a lot of people voice who would have otherwise never been heard from. Some of that has been good, but some of it has been just a real solid pain in the ass. Whatever people say, the AIDS organizations that were formed were good and grew into something great. At some point they will outlive their purpose and reintegrate into the mainstream system of health care or just die off. But their heritage will never deserve denigration.

The actual send-off to Los Angeles was a little more reality-based than my miraculous philosophizing in *The New York Times*. The same group of friends who had helped me the night Joe died plus my good friend Steve Bing came to help pack up the apartment and pack up a truck I had rented to drive myself and my belongings to Los Angeles. I got up early and went downtown to get the truck. Driving in Manhattan in the best of times is a challenge; driving something as big as your apartment is positively thrill-seeking. I hit only one other vehicle between 34th Street and my apartment on West 75th Street. I lived on the seventh floor of my building and we had begun the long and tedious process of getting everything crammed into the small elevator and then out onto the sidewalk. Lamps, chairs, bags of clothing, Joe's ashes housed in two boxes given to me by the funeral home—everything out on the sidewalk. That was when the rain began. It was a light sprinkle at first, a veiled threat really. A light little May shower to dampen my entire world.

I had parked in front of the building entrance on 76th Street on a day that turned out to be garbage-collection day. So when the attendant showed up to ticket me, I put on my best lawyerly skills and went to discuss the matter with him. Garbage trucks, huge New York behemoths, were churning their way down the street. There was no choice, he said, I had to move the truck.

"But I'm moving today." He just looked at me and pulled out his thick book of tickets. "To California," I added as if this would change his mind. It didn't. I got in the truck and started the engine, looking longingly at my possessions lined up on the sidewalk next to the garbage, getting damp in the light rain. "To

California where they don't treat their people this way," I said to Rick as we got in the truck to drive around for a while until the garbage came and went. "Damn right," said Rick.

After a 15-minute drive I went back to the apartment and found it clear of garbage trucks, but now found a huge moving truck, the professional kind, parked near the door where I had been. This was more than inconvenient and meant that, parking behind it, we had to now transport my things down the middle of the block, which was the closest I could park—or rather double-park.

We hurriedly got everything into the truck, but my hopes of an early start had long been shattered by the time we took off at almost noon. I said good-bye to Steve and Tim and Bruce, who thankfully remembered that we needed to tie everything down in the back. I wouldn't have bothered at that point; I would have just taken off and let the chips fall where they might. We drove up Broadway to catch the George Washington Bridge. I drove and Rick sat smoking in the passenger seat. Still getting my sea legs in this mammoth truck, I offended more than a few drivers while Rick leaned out the window yelling at anyone who blew their horn: "Just what New York needs, another critic" or "Yeah, buddy, we're moving to L.A.; we're really gonna miss your ugly face." When we got to the bridge, we sang "California, Here We Come," just as the Ricardos and the Mertzes had in *I Love Lucy*, and it somehow made the challenging morning better. Something tells me we weren't the first fags to do this, but we thought we were.

Once we were in New Jersey it pissed rain. I could barely see where I was going but had enough adrenaline to get us to the western edge of Pennsylvania, the farthest west Rick had ever been. We stopped at a Holiday Inn and had a civilized dinner and stared at the truck in disbelief. I couldn't believe I had done this. Inside that truck was everything—my dead lover, my two cats, all worldly possessions. Behind me, everyone I cared for, and ahead, nothing but the hope that this was the right thing to do.

After seven days and several choruses of *California Dreamin'* with the Mamas and the Papas, we pulled up to the apartment building where I had rented a small apartment that, by New York standards, was pretty wonderful if for no other reasons than it was brand new and it had a dishwasher, neither of which was attainable in New York. We arrived on the day of the expected earthquake, predicted by Nostradamus. We carried the stuff in, waited. Nostradamus, it appeared, had been wrong, so we went to sleep. We spent a fun week exploring L.A., and then Rick had to go home, and I had to go to work.

"Good-bye. Thanks for helping. I love you," I said.

"I love you more," he said

---

Almost immediately the dream that was California gave way to a strong dose of reality. The languid days of enjoying Mike and Allen's hospitality were gone, and there were no more flowers on my breakfast plate. After a hurried bagel and hot coffee, I would drive my 35-mile commute to work where I would be directing a small hospital-based HIV program. When I first showed up for work, I was told that for a new employee a physical was necessary. The last discrimination case I had handled before leaving New York was under a very similar situation, where a man who was an X-ray technician had undergone a physical, and it was revealed in the course of it that he had HIV. The hospital, a major one in New York that should have known better, declined to go ahead with the hiring.

It was a good case for me to make an exit on, if for no other reason than it was nasty and stupid. This was a hospital in New York City, not a convenience store in the Texas panhandle, and the people responsible should have had enough sophistication not to make this kind of mistake in 1987. But in addition the opposing legal counsel was unpleasant to deal with. We finally settled the case this way: If my client could obtain a letter from a doctor stating that he was in fit condition to fulfill the obligations of his job, he would be hired after all. "However," said the little dressed-for-success, yuppie, ivy-league lawyer, "don't think you can just run to one of your doctor friends and have him write it up," she said, looking at me accusingly. I responded that she was hardly in a position to question my ethics, given the nature of the case, and I followed it with a few well-considered expletives.

At any rate I went into my physical with some degree of apprehension. I had to go to Employee Health to do it. Even the name seemed to suggest a threat—Employee Health. If I was HIV-positive, this wasn't the way I wanted to find out, but I was greatly worried that they would bring up my HIV status and ask me to take a test. Even though I knew this to be illegal, I didn't want to sue my new employer. I was fresh out of money after all, 3,000 miles from what I considered to be home, and I needed the job. But during the physical, nothing of this nature came up, and the nurse who was working with me was pleasant enough. She did ask me where I was coming from and what I would be doing at the hospital. I told her I would be directing AIDS outpatient services. We had a pleasant conversation, and then I went back to my office—no discussion of my HIV status. Everything was going to be OK. I told myself how silly I had been to be worrying so much.

Two days later my boss called me to say that there was a problem with my physical. Apparently, the nurse had filed an incident report about our meeting. She stated that while she was taking my history a small speck of saliva had come from my mouth while I was talking and landed right in her eye. She now wanted me to take an HIV test. I told my boss that I would not submit to an HIV test. She explained further that the nurse was two months' pregnant.

There was no way I was going to take this test for this reason, and I made it very clear. I immediately launched into a mild yet firm lawyer-attack mode. "I brought some of the very first AIDS discrimination suits in New York," I said calmly, "and I didn't lose any of them." This wasn't a lie, but the truth is they were administrative proceedings and we always managed to settle them before they went to full hearings. I didn't say anything else. I didn't need to.

While I was calm in my discussions with my employers, I was fairly angry and feeling very threatened. Aside from the fact that I needed the job, I wasn't ready to know my status, not after only having been in California for two weeks. I was incredulous that the nurse would ask me to take an HIV test and that the fact that she was pregnant was supposed to make the outcome of my decision different. What difference did it make what my HIV status was? If my test were negative, how would she know that I hadn't been infected a few months before and wasn't showing antibodies yet. If I had a negative test, did that mean she would worry less? No, she would still have to take her own HIV test. More important, if my test were positive, what did that mean for her? Would she abort her child? No, she'd still have to take her own test. The truth of the matter is no one should ever rely on another person's HIV test results when making a decision. Any way you cut it, she would have to take her own HIV test if she were concerned about that fleck of spit and my test was indicative perhaps but not conclusive.

The next day, the president of the hospital came to my office. He said that he was aware of the misunderstanding and that he hoped that nothing had been misconstrued to imply that an HIV test was being required of me as a condition for my employment. I said that was a great relief to me, and the matter was never spoken of again. But with this episode the Mamas and the Papas lyrics—"California dreamin' is becoming a reality"—had a new slant to the words. Now I knew what reality they were talking about, and I felt a little betrayed. But in fact reality had only begun pissing on my dream.

*42,908 new cases of AIDS were diagnosed*
*27,716 more people died*
*A cumulative total of 149,902 cases were diagnosed*
*89,817 people were dead of AIDS in America*

## A LAPSE IN MEMORY

When I first moved to New York in 1977 a few days after I graduated from college in Illinois, I dated a guy named Carter. He was about seven years older than I was, which seemed very worldly at the time. Our relationship didn't last very long because frankly he wasn't very nice to me, and after a few months we parted company for many years. But almost a decade later we had a chance to become reacquainted when he brought his boyfriend to my office at GMHC for the purpose of getting his will written because he had AIDS. The boyfriend was a very upbeat little guy who made several jokes throughout the process, seemingly in an effort to keep Carter's spirits up.

After I moved to California, Carter's boyfriend died. He called to tell me and to ask if he could come visit me in Los Angeles.

Aware of how important it is to do all those "right things," I said that he could come, though we really hadn't much in common anymore. His visit was pleasant enough. He stayed a week, and we shopped, went to the beach, and took long drives. It was kind of pleasant getting reacquainted under circumstances that didn't involve the pressures of dating.

He left, and we kept in touch by telephone. But one day while we were talking Carter asked me if I was taking my AZT regularly like a good boy. I wondered how and why he made such an obvious mistake and a little chill went up my spine.

"I'm not taking AZT, Carter. I don't have AIDS."

"Oh," he said quietly, considering his mistake. He didn't mention anything else about it, nor did I. I decided that it was just a simple lapse of memory, spooky as it was. But the next time we spoke, the problem appeared more serious. Carter told me that he had gone to his regular therapist appointment at 5:30, but that instead of arriving at 5:30 P.M., he arrived at 5:30 in the morning. Since Carter lived on Staten Island, a trip to Manhattan on the ferry in the wee hours of the morning should have let him know that he was on the wrong track. Clearly, it sounded as if Carter had AIDS dementia, a condition often tossed around by media but of which I had rarely seen or heard of true cases. He related this incident to me rather matter-of-factly without alarm, as if he were telling me that he had just had a bad cold.

I looked at my clock and asked him if he knew that he had called me at 3:30 in the morning.

"No," he said calmly and without apology, "I didn't realize that."

But the next time Carter called, he was crying. I looked at my clock and saw that it was 1:30 A.M., 4:30 in New York.

"Mark," he said, "I have some terrible news."

"What is it Carter?"

"My father died yesterday." Now this was the kind of phone call that was appropriate for the middle of the night. Carter had moved in with his father and was now living in an apartment on the upper east side, the same small apartment in which he had grown up. His mother had been dead for several years.

"I'm so sorry, Carter. What happened? Was he sick? Was this expected?"

"He had a heart attack," he said.

"Are you alone?"

"No," he said, "my brother is staying with me." We talked and he seemed calm and after a while, we rang off. The next day I was surprised when I answered the phone to hear Carter on the other end.

"Mark," he began, "I have terrible news."

"What?"

"It's my father—he died last week."

"He did?" I asked.

"Yes, he had a stroke," he said and began to cry.

A few days later Carter phoned again to tell me that his father had passed away, this time of cancer. What kind of hell is this, I thought; every day Carter gets the sad news that his father died and experiences the same grief and shock all over again, not remembering that the very same thing had happened just the day before. Ever since then I keep debating in my mind whether this was a blessing or a curse. Fortunately, Carter did not have long to suffer this. A few months later his brother called to tell me that Carter was dead.

## NEIL

Neil and I had grown up together in southern Illinois in a small, unattractive town across the Mississippi River from St. Louis called Granite City. We both knew about our sexuality at an early age, 15, and had open discussions about it. We also had very different approaches to it. I was in no hurry to tell my family; he was in a big hurry to tell his. However, the difference in style made neither of us more inclined to stick around home when we came of age. We both went away to school, and the same year we graduated, we headed to the big city. Except his idea of the big city was San Francisco and mine was New York. I've always wondered if the difference between our respective styles could have been summed up by the fact that his parents were conservative Republicans while mine were liberal Democrats.

Neil could never understand why I was so enamored of New York, and while I found San Francisco charming, after a few days there it seemed small to me. He, of course, liked the energy of New York, and most certainly the opportunities such as going to the theater often, but he hated it for being dirty and in his mind, unsafe. For years we kept a constant battle going over whose city was best.

We spoke often on the phone and more and more our conversations turned to the subject of Neil's health. He worked in a testing and counseling center, and so he had tested for HIV relatively early on. I wanted to avoid these conversations for my own testing purposes, and I also didn't want to be faced with the fact that Neil might someday get sick. So until he started becoming ill, I tried vainly to steer the conversation away from talk about HIV.

By the time I moved to Los Angeles, though, Neil was sick. One of the many reasons I was glad to move to the West Coast was that I thought that if he needed me, I would be in much better proximity. He seemed happy with the thought as well, though if there is one place worse than New York in the mind of a San Franciscan, it is Los Angeles, and he couldn't understand why I would move there instead of San Francisco.

I went up to see him as often as time permitted, though in doing so I was aware that one of the less noble reasons I had moved from New York was that I didn't want to watch a whole slew of friends who I knew were sick get sicker and die. So while on the one hand I wanted to be there for Neil; on the other hand I didn't. In most respects, I thought my personal care-taking days were over. Neil had lots of friends and a wonderful lover named Glen.

Neil had developed a disease called *Mycobacterium avium* intracellulare. As I understood it, it acted almost like a systemic tuberculosis. Symptoms included some nausea but also a gnawing fatigue. The thing about MAI is that it used to be fairly rare as an opportunistic infection. People usually got diagnosed with it when they were at the very end of the disease spectrum. However, the unusual thing in Neil's case was that it was the first opportunistic infection with which he was diagnosed. The very worst thing about MAI, however, was that the only treatment for it was highly experimental and seemed to have endless side effects that were almost worse than anything the disease offered up. In 1989 I drove up to have Thanksgiving with Neil and his family, who had come in to see him. He was having a very hard time physically. He had always been skinny, but now he was very thin. He had never given up smoking, and he looked more like a cancer patient than a person with AIDS. We had a very nice dinner together, which since I love to cook, I found therapeutic.

A few months later Neil was worse. I went up to see him. He was very thin. He was having difficulty with a number of bodily functions, and it was humiliating for him. He cried some of the time, but he also yelled. He was really angry. I sat in his bed and held him for a while before I left. He was so upset; I told him I would come back in ten days for another visit. The following week Glen called to tell me that Neil had been to the doctor and was told that he was going to die soon and that nothing could be done to help him. He said that Neil came home so distressed that after telling Glen about the trip to the doctor, he lay down and went to sleep. Then Neil went into a coma. His family was called, and they had went to San Francisco. Then he told me that Neil was dead.

The next day I drove up to San Francisco through hot desert. When I got into the city it was freezing cold. I pulled up to this house around 3 in the afternoon, and his whole family was there to greet me and hug me. They decided they would want dinner in and asked if I would prepare something. Everyone wanted something different, so I made swordfish and softshell crabs. Getting a dinner for several people together in short order was arduous. It involved going to do the marketing, setting up in a strange kitchen and doing your best to make it a good dinner de spite the way everyone feels.

Neil's family had always been strictly nonalcoholic. Mine was not. While cooking, I was pulling the cork out of a wine bottle when Neil's mother appeared at the kitchen door. She looked surprised and said, "What are you doing?"

"Well," I said as the cork popped, "I'm having a glass of wine because, frankly, I need one." She just stood there looking at me, still with that somewhat surprised expression on her face.

"Would you like to join me?" I ventured.

"Yes, I think I'll have a little glass." I turned down all the burners and poured us two glasses. We sat and talked quietly at the kitchen table about all of this and how unfair it was. Neil's sister Jan appeared at the door and later told me in tears that Neil would have been so happy to see his mom having that glass of wine.

The next day we had the memorial service for Neil. He had many friends and as part of the service, we all went up to the front of the room and signed a quilt panel that had been hurriedly assembled. Each of us wrote something to Neil on it. I signed my name just under his and wondered for the umpteenth time how long it would be before I would have one of these of my own.

## BUDDY TO THE STARS

Several months after moving to L.A., I was reading in bed late one night when my telephone rang. I looked at the clock and wondered who could be calling at the late hour.

"Hello?"

"Hi, Mark Senak?"

"Yep."

"This is Brad Davis. Do you remember me?"

Well, I wanted to say, "Gee, no Brad, I don't remember you. I had countless fantasies about you from the time I saw you in *Midnight Express* kissing another man on the lips, the very first time I saw that on the screen. Or there could be the time I sat beside you in a New York restaurant. Or let me see, there could be the time that Rodger McFarlane introduced us backstage after one of the several performances of *The Normal Heart* that I sat through. Or if I still didn't remember you, there was the time I was walking down the street, delirious from shopping for a new Speedo that I was going to wear on a weekend trip to California because Joe was feeling better and I needed a break. That night you were walking down Greenwich with Larry Kramer and the two of you were having a knock-down drag-out full-fledged screaming argument about something. Larry stopped and said hello and reintroduced us. Larry tried to drag me into the argument and decide who was right, and I could only respond by saying that I had just bought a new bathing suit and was off to California the next day, and I didn't really care who was right. Hmm, Brad...Brad Davis, am I right? Little guy? Weren't you in *Chariots of Fire*?"

But Brad's voice sounded so small on the phone. He sounded so frightened that I knew that this was one of the few situations of my life where sarcasm didn't seem appropriate.

"Sure, Brad, I remember you."

"Rodger said I could talk to you and that I could trust you."

"Well, if Rodger said that, it must be true," I said, impressed with my snappy comeback despite the fact that I was feeling a little intimidated.

"I have HIV."

It was pretty impressive, I thought, that a man who sounded so frightened came right out with that. He told me that he found out that he was HIV-positive while filming something in Italy. He had donated blood at Cedars-Sinai, and they had sent a letter to his home. His wife had read it to him over the phone. So much for confidentiality procedures.

"Not the best way to get that sort of news," I said. "What's your status now, have you been sick at all?"

"No, but I don't feel as energetic as I did. I need to see a doctor."

"You won't go to your own doctor?"

"I won't go to any doctor."

"Well, I can make some calls and get you into an office after-hours somewhere."

"No, I won't go to an office."

"Well, you are better off in the office. Hollywood isn't exactly teeming with doctors who make house calls you know."

"No!" he said. "I won't go to a doctor's office." This was our first of what would be many disagreements. "If someone sees me or sees my medical record, I won't be working anymore. I need to work. I have a family."

"Well, I'll need to think about how to do this," I said. "Can we talk again tomorrow?"

"Yeah, sure. I'd like to meet you."

Brad kept me on the phone for about 45 minutes that night. He was deeply in need of reassurance that I was someone he could trust. He told me that only a few people knew of his diagnosis, his wife, his manager, his shrink, Rodger, Larry Kramer, and now me. We talked until I felt that I really needed to go to sleep and told him I'd talk to him the next day. I hung up and pulled the blankets over me and felt sorry for how very frightened he was. I wondered how he lived with so much fear, without thinking about the fact that for the past several years almost everyone I knew was afraid. The fear just took on a different form for people. I went to sleep that night wondering if this was the kind of happenstance I would often come across in my new life in Hollywood.

Other than doing legal work for people with AIDS and being Joe's full-time support, I had never volunteered as an HIV "buddy." But now I was enlisted and, yes, I was partly starstruck, but I don't know a gay man who wouldn't be. But it was impossible to not be touched by this man's very human need and above all by his almost tangible fear. Brad needed more than a doctor referral; he needed someone he could call and talk to. In my world AIDS was a global thing, but in Brad's it was narrowed to a small circle of people he could trust.

He did call the next day but only to talk, again needing to get comfortable with the idea he had just told me his deepest secret and made himself so vulnerable to someone he didn't even know. Later that week we met at City restaurant at about 5:30. It would become our regular meeting spot. It was at Second

Street and La Brea and not far from where I was living. The first time we met I went home from work and changed clothes five times. I ordered a martini; Brad ordered water. I felt like a lush. Brad didn't drink.

Apparently he used to, along with other recreational indulgences, the details of which I never asked. I didn't care. We weren't too much into talking about the past; we were mostly interested in what he could do in the future. That first meeting was just a get-acquainted thing. We sat at a table near the front, and there was almost no one else there, since it was so early in the afternoon. Brad let me know right away, before I embarrassed myself, how much it bugged him to be remembered for his role in *Midnight Express* and nothing else. Not long after that some guy came in and sat a few tables away. He had long blond hair and a vacant dazed look that fixed on Brad.

"Hey, hey," he said pointing at Brad. "Billy Hayes, am I right?" Brad looked at him and resignedly said, "Yep." Then we got up and moved tables to one at the other end of the empty restaurant.

Brad got his medical care because Rodger, who now worked at Broadway Cares, made some calls and arranged for a well-known HIV physician to see Brad at his home. There was a doctor who made house calls after all. Brad couldn't say enough wonderful things about the doctor. Brad began to ask endless questions about HIV. People with HIV are more activist and knowledgeable about their condition than any other disease-specific group and know more about their treatment options. But Brad was different; he was still on the outside looking in, and I was surprised that I had never met anyone with HIV who knew so little about it.

One day we met at City for drinks. Well, I met for drinks. Brad had just had a T-cell test. "How many?" I asked, hopeful. He looked so damn happy, I thought the news must be good.

"Well, I called in and they told me 143." He was grinning from ear to ear because this sounded like a lot to him. I'm sitting there knowing that anything below 200 lays a person open to having a whole host of opportunistic infections that can kill and can certainly cause a lot of pain. I'm sitting there knowing that most people in this range have what used to be called full-blown AIDS. Brad sees a cloud pass over me, a look of uncertainty in my eyes. He senses my disappointment with the instincts of a hunting dog, not that it would take one. "One hundred forty-three," he says again, "that's good isn't it?"

At this point I imagine that my head is like one of those eight balls from the 1960s that you ask a question and turn over and the answer floats to the top. Every time I lie, the word LIE floats to the top of my forehead for everyone to see.

He stared at my face. "That's good, isn't it?" The words sound so small and pleading.

I paused. I want to find a way to make this good. I smoothed out the already smooth table cloth. "Good is relative," I said. "The numbers game isn't such a good one to play." Brilliant. Now he was completely upset. His eyebrows came together, and he looked so very afraid. I felt responsible, as if I had made his T-cell count fall so low. "Look, I know people with four T cells who have never been sick, and I know people with 300 who feel like shit. I don't think T cells are necessarily what it's all about." Brad just sat there looking as if I'd hit him in the face. I ordered a martini.

That was pretty much the way it was. In essence, I became Brad's buddy. When the epidemic began, people had a need for two kinds of services—one, they needed information because no one knew anything about what was causing this new, awful disease; and second, they needed emotional support because it was so hideously awful and people treated them in an awful way. Most AIDS service organizations responded by creating a hotline for people to call for information and a buddy program to lend emotional and practical support. Buddies got assigned to a person and passed time with him until his client died. They went to movies, helped out around the house, helped run errands. Basically they were what the name said they were—they were buddies. I was Brad's buddy.

*48,564 new cases of AIDS were diagnosed*
*31,438 more people died*
*A cumulative total of 198,466 cases were diagnosed*
*121,255 people were dead of AIDS in America*

## CHEAP SENTIMENT

What began as a late-night phone call from a kind of desperate guy grew into one of the nicest friendships of my life. I grew to care about Brad a great deal, and he cared about me. We did the usual things friends did, though City restaurant was always sort of our home base and regular hangout. Sometimes we went to Dupar's and had breakfast in the middle of the day, but that was a demanding thing because Brad would eat pancakes and drink diet Coke in front of me, and that was a little hard to watch in the middle of the day.

One day he called with a sense of urgency. He had a chance at a film role, but the shoot would be in Italy. What would happen if a search of his luggage would find his AZT and other medications, he asked. What are the rules of foreign countries about admitting people with HIV. I tried to explain to him that the United States, perhaps the greatest exporter of HIV in the world, had one of the more restrictive policies and that Italy shouldn't be a problem. But Brad wanted definite answers to specific questions about which he had very strong fears.

He wasn't always filled with fear and urgency, though. There was the part of Brad that needed a friend like me with whom he could talk about HIV, but there was also the side of Brad who liked to have fun with his friends. People who are familiar with Brad's acting career would perceive an utterly serious, no-nonsense heavy on the machismo little dynamo of a marine type of guy. *Midnight Express* and *Querelle* each had tough street types. But one thing missed in all those performances was his sense of humor and his really comic side.

"You should do more comedy," I said after seeing *Rosalie Goes Shopping*. "Your timing is really good."

"Tell that to my agent!" he screamed in my ear.

Brad knew that I had a phobia of rats in movie theaters. This developed in New York as a consequence of an incident during my viewing of the movie *Gallipoli*. At the very climactic close of the film, just as the tension has built to a crescendo and we are to find out if the hero, played by Mel Gibson, dies or stays alive on a hopeless mission, a person in the front of the theater yelled, "Oh, my God, rats!" There was a panicked murmur all over the theater, and within a few seconds the feet of the entire audience went up in the air. It was like trying to watch the movie through a forest of legs. I missed the entire end of the movie. I went back a few days later to a different theater and saw it again. It makes sense that rats would congregate in movie theaters with those nice sticky floors littered with so many tasty food items. So from that day on I always wore high-topped shoes to the movies, never sandals. I told Brad this story and he, like many of my friends, thought I was crazy.

We were in Beverly Hills seeing *Cinema Paradiso*. About a fourth of the way through the film, I heard a noise. It was the kind of sound a rat would make. I turned and looked at Brad, slumped down in his seat watching the English subtitles. I leaned over and whispered, "Did you hear that."

"Sh-h-h!" He was angry. He was so serious about movies and art. You didn't interrupt art to talk. I went back to reading subtitles, and I heard the noise again. I started to ask Brad if he had heard that noise, but he shushed me again, this time more annoyed. So I tried to ignore it, but I was unnerved. I stopped eating my popcorn and listened in the dark. Then, I felt it brush up against my ankle. I shivered and jumped, trying not to shriek so that I didn't cause a panic in the theater. I didn't want to ruin *Cinema Paradiso* the way *Gallipoli* had been ruined. I didn't want to interrupt anyone's art. I didn't want a rat on me either. I was sitting with my knees to my chest and my feet off the ground trying to see my loathsome enemy on the floor, leering at me, greedily going after popcorn I had dropped. Brad was smiling. Then Brad was laughing. He stuck out his lips and made his rat noise and then brushed his hand against my elevated ankle. I couldn't believe it. Mr. Serious Art was interrupting my movie enjoyment, my movie viewing, *my* art. I tried to scold him, but all it got me was another "Sh-h-h!" and everyone looked at me. When we got outside I threw this whole episode in his face, and he told me I was crazy. I pointed out to him that it was very hypocritical, and he told me I was neurotic. It was one of many fights we enjoyed having.

We fought a lot. It was never serious, though anyone who would have overheard us would have thought we were locked in an eternal version of the Bickersons. Later, after his death, when I spoke at Brad's memorial service, held at the Doolittle Theater in Hollywood, I said that I would miss our arguments. After I sat down, Brad's wife, Susan, turned to me and said, "Brad loved to fight with you too."

The subject of a fight never mattered. It was the sport of it. Once in City we somehow got to arguing about animal testing. Brad asked me how I can buy products from companies that engage in animal testing—"making rabbits go blind to test mascara."

"Well," I said, "they make rabbits go blind testing mascara so that second-rate actors don't go blind when they wear it in second-rate films." I thought for a minute I had gone too far. All conversation stopped, and he never took his eyes off me. In a gesture that made me think more of Margo Channing than Brad Davis, he placed a hand up to his neck and lowered his chin and eyelashes. "I *never* wore mascara."

The way I've described a buddy would lend the impression that it is a one-sided relationship, with the buddy helping out the "victim." But Brad was as much my buddy as I was his. One of our biggest arguments was about my hypocrisy on one point. It was now 1990, and I still had never taken an HIV antibody test. Brad was absolutely incredulous.

"It's so fuckin' hypocritical of you to work for an organization that tells people to take the test, and you tell people to take the test, and you yourself won't take it."

"That isn't quite the situation," I would say, embarrassed nonetheless. "Taking a test is a very personal decision. It isn't something someone else decides for you. I don't tell people they should take the test; I encourage them to do it."

"You sound like a lawyer."

"I am a lawyer."

"You are a hypocrite."

And that is the way that argument went. It only ended when I was able to distract him with some other issue that we had argued about—so we wouldn't stop arguing, we'd just change tracks. Sometimes, though, he was like a dog with a bone.

"Look, Brad," I would try to explain, "an HIV test does not occur in a medical vacuum. It's not just a test for antibodies; it's a test of every system in your life. It's a test of your insurance, your job status, your relationships with your family and loved ones. It's a test of everything on which you rely. I'm just not ready to do that."

When Brad and I first connected in Los Angeles, I was still working at the medical center, where I hadn't been very happy. Two very good things came from that job, though. The first was meeting a coworker, Kate Graber, who became then and still is one of my best friends. It is one of those friendships that comes from the unlikely venue of a workplace and blossoms into something lifelong. The other was that my duties had brought me into frequent contact with AIDS Project Los Angeles, the second largest AIDS service organization in the country after GMHC. Switching jobs, I didn't want a pre-existing condition documented before I entered a new group insurance program. Then if I got sick, I wouldn't be covered.

"Well," said Brad, happy to be enlightening me for a change, "you could test anonymously."

"I could, but what use is the information if I'm not going to medically intervene. Once I know I'm HIV-positive, I need to get T-cell counts, I need to begin documenting that condition in my medical record. Once that's done, I am locked in my job because of insurance reasons. This isn't a medical test, Brad."

"But there are things you can do now, medicines to take."

"What? AZT? I've watched the AZT thing, and while it has some impact, it is not really amounting to anything other than postponing the inevitable." That was a hard thing to say to someone who was HIV-positive, and I wouldn't have said it but for the fact that he was so adamant, so strident that I needed to be tested. I couldn't say it to him, but after all, he had to think AZT was great. He had no choice; he was taking it.

"So," he said, obviously hurt by that last comment, "then you can add time."

"Longevity," I said flatly, "is not necessarily my goal. Why does everyone think that he who lives the longest wins? I'm not about seeing how long I can live."

Then a rare thing from Brad: sentiment. "I want you to take the test because I care about you."

Not fair. Hitting below the belt.

"I adore cheap sentiment," I said.

This was sort of the discussion we had about a dozen times, in various forms. Sometimes he would get heated up; sometimes he just spoke out of quiet concern. But I wasn't ready to do this for practical reasons, and I was also not ready to do this emotionally. I would lie awake at night and relive every sexual instance in my life that could have facilitated transmission of HIV. For me, sex was usually in the context of dating, and frankly, I hadn't dated that many men. And actually, I reasoned, if you listened to the science on transmission, there weren't many possibilities for me. HIV is spread by blood-to-blood contact, by semen-to-blood contact, through the birth canal, or ingested during breastfeeding. I had had no blood-to-blood contact and obviously no birth issues, which only left semen-to-blood.

In the early 1980s Todd and I had not been safe. No one had. And while I hadn't gotten sick, that was no guarantee that I hadn't been infected. But the good news was that Todd was also still alive, at least he had been when I ran into him in at the quilt display in Washington in 1987. But that had been three years ago, an entire lifetime in AIDS terms.

Then there was and is the entire debate about oral transmission of HIV. At each and every international AIDS conference, I saw several posters from European sources saying that oral sex was not a high-risk activity. Posters from the United States, cast doubts on that assertion. It has never been a well-defined area. Well, that leaves a range of open possibilities, and as a gray area left a nice large gray hole in any sense of security I might have about my comparatively conservative sexual practices.

## SWEAT IT OUT, BABY

I had heard about night sweats over the years. They are a symptom that something is wrong, seriously wrong, and they can be a symptom of an upcoming bout of pneumocystis pneumonia. In the early years of the epidemic, pamphlets contained descriptions of the warning signs of AIDS—shortness of breath, swollen glands, night sweats. That is why in the middle of the night in the spring of 1990, when I woke up in a bed at 3 A.M. completely soaked with sweat, I knew that there was no question—I was dying.

Night sweats had often been described. "The bed is soaked. You can literally wring the sheets out." I thought these to be exaggerations of waking up and finding you were sweating badly. They aren't exaggerations. I did wring out my sheets, which were cold and damp as if it had rained inside the apartment. The bed, once stripped of its linens, had a large oval wet stain, bigger than the outline of my body. It was too wet to make up again, so I left the sheets off and went and lay down on the couch and thought about my upcoming death. I decided I would take treatment for this bout of pneumocystis and buy enough time to wrap up my life. I wondered if I should go home to my family to die or just stay here in California. Why, oh why, I thought, had I left New York? There, people would be around to help me and I wouldn't feel isolated by having this disease. Here, I hadn't made too many friends and still only had Michael and my friend Kate, who would do anything for me. Three in the morning is such a vulnerable time. Demonic images you would otherwise dismiss outright come forth with a dramatic presence and a strength that takes advantage of your tired, sleepy self. I spent the rest of the night lying on my couch trying to make decisions about my life with what was left of it.

The next day at work I decided to tell no one what had happened. But my nerves were not up to that, and I told a nurse who was on my staff. She helped me with my denial. There can be lots of reasons for night sweats, she said. But neither of us thought of any. I got busy with the day and didn't think much about what had happened until later when it came time for me to go to bed. The bed was still damp and couldn't be made up. I couldn't even pretend that it hadn't happened with the evidence staring me in the face like that. I would have to sleep on the couch. I did decide to call Brad and tell him what had happened, knowing that he would pressure me into getting an HIV test.

Brad listened as I told him what had happened. "That's it, then," he said. "You have to go get tested." I think I called Brad to test myself, to see if he could convince me to do that which I knew I should be doing in the first place.

"Look," I said, "my doctor has been trying different kinds of blood-pressure medication because it's been high. Maybe it is just a side effect of that, you know, like my blood pressure did something weird during the night."

"Yeah, so then you go to the doctor and you find out what is going on and get the fucking test."

I hung up no more or less convinced than I had been before, but by the following morning after having spent the night on the floor, I noticed that the damp spot appeared gone. That sort of settled it for me. I made up the bed. Getting rid of this physical reminder would help make the problem go away. I was in a hurry to get to work, so that I would be distracted. I was able to push back the dark thoughts of the imminent horrors that waited for me. I no longer felt compelled to thoroughly examine my body for any unexpected bruise-type marks that might be there. I wondered if I could get my favorite doctor at work to give me my bronchoscopy, that unpleasant procedure in which a tube is shoved down one's nasal passages and throat to the lungs in order to diagnose pneumocystis pneumonia. They're gonna have to give me a ton of Valium was all I could think. Those were my thoughts yesterday, but today I was going to treat the whole thing for what it was—a fluke.

It worked. I began to pretend as if the incident hadn't occurred at all. Sometimes there is a fine line between denial and cognitive therapy. By the end of the next day I was showing no other symptoms and did not have any spiking fevers. Whatever had caused the sweats, it wasn't AIDS. After that second day without any symptoms, I went back to sleeping in my bed finally letting go of the obsessive thoughts that had sat on my shoulder like a conscience. I fell asleep, relaxed, letting go, feeling utterly safe.

When I awoke a few hours later at 3 A.M., I was soaked to the skin in wet, cold sheets. It was worse than the first time. I lay in my wet bed, and with what water I had left in my body, I cried.

The next day I called Brad and told him what had happened and told him that I had made an appointment with my doctor.

I had to throw in the towel after almost ten years of wondering about my HIV status. Within the last three days the entire equation was changed. Brad was right: The point had been reached where I needed to know, just for the sake of knowing. It wasn't as if there was treatment I was eager to seek; it was that I couldn't go on living the way I had, as if I were a walking time bomb that would one day explode with enough illness to fill a medical dictionary. Yes, by that time there was AZT and a sister drug, ddI, but their only benefit was to postpone the inevitable in my estimation. What could be the point in that, I thought?

My doctor and I made a deal that allowed me to take the test in her office without it being documented. The results would not go into my medical chart but would be torn up. When I went into her office I felt as if I were stepping onto a space shuttle and blasting off; the whole experience seemed so surreal to me. The nurse drawing the blood told me to relax, that "everything was going to be OK."

This was a nice sentiment. But nothing would ever be OK again. I'd lost too many friends and would lose too many more to ever feel like everything was OK. I spared her this lecture, though, and offered a weak smile of thanks in exchange. I had the constant feeling that I wanted to throw up, especially as she went through the rote of information about when I could expect results. You should know in about a week, she said, maybe sooner.

I knew what that statement meant. A negative test appeared right away, but one that was positive would mean that it would have to be confirmed by a second, more-involved test, and that would take more time. That night I went to bed wondering if the sweats would return. As I fell asleep, I thought about my vial of blood, picked up that day and taken to some laboratory in Southern California. I imagined it on some centrifuge, or whatever happens, while a studious and serious-looking person in a white lab coat looked on impassively, overseeing the answer to my life-and-death question. I fell asleep late.

The next day I had a conference to go to down near Laguna. In the afternoon I was going to be giving a talk at the conference, but I was on automatic pilot, almost unaware of the fact that I was waiting for these test results. There was just that nag-

ging lump in my stomach that wouldn't go away, and I pretended that it wasn't there. I drove down to Orange County and
went through the morning distracting myself by hanging out
with a cute guy I met once I got there. I don't know how I was
able to keep up a conversation, but I did it. Ten minutes before
my talk I called my office and spoke to the office assistant, Mary.

"Any calls?"

"No," said Mary through a rich Jamaican accent, "no one
called."

My heart sank. I thought if there had been a negative result,
my doctor might have called even though that wasn't what we
had talked about.

"Oh," said Mary, "your doctor did call."

"Was there a message."

"They want you to call."

I didn't even say good-bye to Mary but hung up and called
my doctor's office. Being put on hold while they fetched her, I
began to say a delirious prayer. She came on the line.

"Mark?"

"What happened?"

"Everything is OK," she said.

"Thank you, thank you, thank you," I said as if she were responsible for the test result.

"We told you it would be OK." Even in my near delirium, I
had to wonder if 'I told you so' was entirely necessary. I hung up
and began to cry. Headed to the bathroom, I was told that the
room was ready for my talk.

"Tell them I'll be a minute; I'm having contact lens trouble."
I went in the john and cried, and then I threw up. I went out

ten minutes later and waded through my talk. As soon as it was over, I got into my car to drive back to Los Angeles on Interstate 405. Today when I pass that way, I still call to mind driving a particular stretch near Long Beach and gagging as I drove, retching over the side of my car. Fortunately, I had a convertible so everyone who wanted to could see this. Throughout the drive I continued to cry. I thought about Joe and my dead friends. I thought about the enormity of my relief. I wondered why my friends had to die and why I got to live. I wondered if Joe and Neil were somewhere where they could feel my relief, my guilt, and my happiness all at once, just the way I was feeling it. I thought that my life would never be the same. And you know what? It wasn't.

Maybe everything could be OK.

## THE POSITIVE WITH THE NEGATIVE

That night I called my closest friends and let them know. I called Rick Croll, who cried with me on the phone. I thought it might be awkward telling Rick, who was getting pretty sick himself. "Hi, I know you're sick and dying, but I get to live, isn't that wonderful?" Of course that isn't what I said, but it's what it felt like I was saying. His voice was raspy, and I could tell he was having trouble breathing. But he could only sound happy for me, and I was greatly relieved.

I had more hesitation before calling Brad, though. He had known me for less time, and he was struggling against his HIV in a way that Rick wasn't. He was not only afraid of what was going to happen to his health but about his ability to work and risk of the news being public. I tried to downplay the news when I called.

"I found out my test results today. It was negative," I said as quietly as I could. There was a long pause. I wondered if Brad had decided beforehand that I was going to be HIV-positive and was now surprised to find that I wasn't. Was he anticipating having my support not just as friend he could talk to about his own HIV but as a friend in the same boat?

"That's really good news, Mark." His voice was subdued. Then he said, "You don't know how lucky you are." I had nothing to say to that. Somehow I felt that an inevitable gulf would open up between me and Brad. He was sick and I was well, and now no matter how sympathetic and empathetic I wanted to be, I would never know precisely how he felt. That was when I learned what many other HIV-negative men learned; we were embarrassed about being negative, as if we had somehow abandoned our brothers.

Not long after that I got a call from Rick. He had been in the hospital with another bout of pneumocystis, and he wasn't doing so well. He was now living at home with his parents in New Jersey. Once when I called to see how he was doing, his Dad had answered the phone. We had never met, but he knew we were close friends. "Listen," he said, "if you want to see Rick again, I'd do it soon." I knew that it must be bad then if his father knew that Rick had gotten The Look.

My next trip east was scheduled a few weeks later, and I arranged to go out to his parents' house for a visit. I came up from Washington, D.C., and then took a bus from New York out to the small town where they lived. It was a very pleasant spot.

Rick's dad picked me up at the bus station and drove me to their home. When I got there I was shocked to see that once robust Rick was now thin and frail. He came to hug me, and I was a little afraid I'd hurt him. He could barely breathe, and he carried along with him a portable oxygen unit, not unlike the one Joe once had. Clear tubing, from which he drew the oxygen, led up from the small tank and went around Rick's head like a halo that had fallen down below his nose.

"Look, I have a little friend," he said, lifting up the tank. "Makes it nasty when I smoke." Then he gagged laughing at his own joke.

I pretended like this was the most natural thing in the world. I looked at Rick's face. In addition to having lost a great deal of weight, Rick's temples had sunk in. Temporal wasting was one of the surest signs of The Look.

"Well," he said, "I've lost weight with the AIDS diet plan." We gave this the small laugh it deserved. His parents left us alone while Rick gave me a tour of the house. The garden and yard were quite beautiful and lush. It was a nice place to come and die, I thought. That night his parents made dinner out on the grill, and we ate corn on the cob and fresh tomatoes. Rick drank an Ensure, farting and burping. We sat up late and talked about old friends; who was alive, who was dead? I told him that I had run into someone on the street in New York who greeted me by saying, "I thought you were dead." We gossiped and rehashed old stories and laughed at them like we were hearing them for the very first time. We did Bette Davis imitations. We talked about Lucy and Ethel. Nothing had changed. Then Rick had to go to bed, and his mother and I stayed up late and talked. She told me about the many support opportunities there were for them and that the local HIV organization had been very helpful. Rick also had a home attendant who really seemed to help. At some points during our conversation I wondered if she was looking to me to contradict the inevitable. Parents often do that. They say things like, "Well, they're making a lot of progress in research, aren't they?" I've learned through much experience to offer quiet reinforcements, such as "Well, we can certainly hope." But the truth was, there wasn't much hope, and I knew it. But I didn't think it my place to make them know it.

My bus back to the city left the next afternoon. Rick went with me and his dad in the car to the station where I would pick it up. We both knew that this was the last time we would ever see each other. We stood and hugged for a long time, and by some minor miracle neither of us was giving in to tears, even though I could feel my insides turning out.

"I love you," I said.

"I love you more," he said.

Rick's father didn't make it. He stood off to the side and cried like a baby. I waved good-bye through the bus window, and Rick and his dad helped each other back to the car. A few months later Rick's parents called to tell me that he had died.

## GMHC ALL OVER AGAIN

It was July 1990 when I got the much welcomed job offer as director of client services at AIDS Project Los Angeles. When I had left New York I told David Margolick from *The New York Times* that I was going to California to "retire" from AIDS work and that I was going to look for that feeling of renewed hope I had as a kid. But the epidemic was growing so fast that there never seemed to be a time when I could do that. The offer from APLA seemed very natural to me when it came along. It seemed like it was the place I belonged, so I went. There, like at GMHC, I met people who were braver than they knew for the most part. And as director of client services, I was able to put to use some of what I had learned at GMHC about human nature in the face of the epidemic.

There is no question that there was a dedication among my coworkers to their clients. It also becomes apparent how individual each person's experience is with this epidemic and how extremely personal it becomes. APLA was not about a job for any of us. It was about our lives.

As director of client services, I administered several programs that ranged from a dental clinic to legal services to mental health services. I learned a lot, and while I was director, the programs doubled in size and capacity over a two-year period, and I went from having a staff of 45 to one of 90 and a budget that went from about $2.5 million to $5 million and clients that just kept coming and coming and coming.

But there was a difference from GMHC. The clients who came each day for services were poorer than the ones of the day before. They had less formal education than the others. And they were less insured than their predecessors. More and more it became apparent for a growing number of the population we served, AIDS was not their number one problem. They were chronically homeless, substance-addicted, or mentally ill—or sometimes a combination of all three. Ironically and pathetically, for some, AIDS would be the best thing that ever happened to them because if they hadn't had AIDS, there would have been no system of care for them at all. That sad reality makes the dedication of the people who work and volunteer at APLA so different in nature from the workers of the previous decade at GMHC. The world got easier in some ways as AIDS became more accepted and got the support of mainstream institutions such as hospitals. But it got harder when faced with these new challenges. That's what AIDS has been for the people who work with it all these years—one large mass of complicated challenges coming unraveled with each new development or event, like the rubber bands wound up tight inside a golf ball.

---

*59,284 new cases of AIDS were diagnosed*
*36,382 more people died*
*A cumulative total of 257,750 cases were diagnosed*
*157,637 people were dead of AIDS in America*

---

In the summer of 1991 I went to my first international conference on AIDS, held in Florence, Italy. I flew all day and all night, originally scheduled to land in Rome but could only get to Milan at the last moment. Unable to sleep on airplanes, I fell asleep immediately on the train from Milan to Florence. With only a few hours of sleep, I attended the opening ceremonies. AIDS took on new dimensions for me at that conference. There was so much going on all over the world, certainly there would have to be a break soon. But one of the things you discover at a conference like this is not only all of the science we know but all of the science we have yet to learn. The Florence conference was scary if for no other reason than it seemed that there were still mysteries about modes of transmission, particularly around oral sex, a controversy not settled by later conferences.

But one moment of that conference stands out. On the first day on my way to the opening plenary session, I walked across a bridge that connected one side of a busy thoroughfare with another to get to the hall where the session would be held. Below, a large group of angry demonstrators with brightly colored banners stopped traffic and blew whistles. Demonstrations at an AIDS conference are not rare, and in fact in Vancouver in 1996 they would be orchestrated as part of the program. But I had not seen many yet, and I stopped on the bridge to look down at the activity. My passing interest turned to anger when I realized the group was protesting the use of animals in lab experiments for HIV research. I turned away and walked to the hall with my hands balled up in fists and a fast rising anger that overtook me to the point where I was talking to myself. I simply could not believe the affront of this. I loved animals, I loved my animals, but I knew that I'd happily slay every animal I ever met for just ten minutes with almost any of my lost friends.

## THE SECRET IS OVER

Brad and I hadn't seen each other for several weeks at the end of the summer in 1991. He had been sick, and when he went into the hospital, which he entered under an assumed name, he specifically told me by telephone not to visit him. He did not want me to see him while he was sick, he said. I thought that my seeing him in any sort of semihelpless position would be difficult for both of us. Patient was not a role I thought he would play well. He came out of the hospital and was apparently terribly unhappy and feeling ill. He went back in a second time and then returned home. Rodger was going to let me know when he was feeling better.

On the following Monday morning I was about to go into a staff meeting when Mike Lombardo called me.

"Is it true about Brad Davis?" he asked.

"Is what true?" I said slowly, not used to discussing this with anyone outside our circle.

"Brad Davis died."

I had grown accustomed to words uttered on a phone telling me that I had lost a friend. But under most circumstances I expected it. My friends had been sick, and we all knew that death was near and that the phone call would come at any time. But when Mike uttered these words, it was like I'd been kicked in the stomach.

I went into my meeting thinking that it couldn't be true. I didn't speak during the entire meeting, not uncommon for me, since I hated them. But it was a long wait to get out of the meeting and get the news confirmed, which I did by calling Rodger. Brad had died the night before. We didn't get to say good-bye.

On Wednesday the *Los Angeles Times* carried a full story on the front page of the Metro section about the ordeal Brad had been through in trying to keep his secret and his career. It talked about our small circle who had kept Brad's secret. The board chair of APLA called me to say he was sorry and then asked me how many other secrets I was harboring. Because of Brad's fear of the Hollywood Establishment, the media had a lot of questions about the secret we had kept for so long. It was terribly difficult to talk about, not only because I was sad that Brad died but also because I was so used to guarding the secret so closely for so long. I had never told my family or my best friends, and I felt as if I was betraying Brad by talking about it at all even though everyone else was talking about it. The fact that word was out was slow to sink in. Trying to talk about it was like finding I could speak a foreign language without having ever spoken it before. My mouth wrapped around the words "Brad" and "AIDS" in the same sentence only with the greatest reluctance.

Having read the newspaper, Peter Jennings's office from ABC called me and asked if they could speak to Susan, Brad's wife. I called her and relayed for a bit between the two. ABC lost patience when I hesitated, and the producer who called me said, "Look, we have her number; we can call her at any time. We're dealing through you out of respect for her privacy." They along with everyone else finally interviewed her. Susan and I only met at the memorial service for the first time, though we had spoken several times on the phone. She is a lovely and loving woman.

The media frenzy was immediate, fast, and furious. Within a few days of the story in the *Times*, Susan and I did a talk show together telling and retelling our story that for so long we had kept a secret. What bothered me most of all, however, was the level of prurient interest exhibited not only by media but by people I knew. Everyone asked me questions about "how" Brad got HIV. I never knew. I never asked him. I never cared. But in all the asking, no one asked me whether Brad suffered a great deal. No one asked about his illness. Everyone asked how he got it. I was so disappointed in everyone, and I felt bitter about it. My growing disenchantment with the media only grew when ABC had hinted that they might pick Brad as the ABC News

Person of the Week. Instead, that Friday when I watched, the Person of the Week was Blondie Bumstead, the cartoon-strip character, because in the comic strip she was finally going to get a job. Wow.

There was one other secret still kept. Brad died because he chose to. He took something that killed him; the MAI did not do it. When I was told this on the day after he died, I was so stunned. I have always been an advocate for people in this situation, and I have never thought they should be second-guessed by the community of people who are well. Their decision, I've always argued, is between themselves and God. We are certainly entitled to our opinions, but we really have no right to judge them until we are lying in that bed with cancer or some form of chronic, awful, and terminal pain. If someone wants out earlier, it is up to him, not to us.

But that firmly held conviction held up like toilet paper when I got the news that Brad had killed himself, because despite my overwhelming sentiment on the matter, when I got the news, it wasn't about Brad—it was about me. I was so angry. How could he do that? There were still things that might be done. He might have had months and months of quality life. What if they found an effective treatment soon? And most of all, he didn't even say good-bye. All my words about longevity not being my goal came back to haunt me. The anger passed, and compassion and reason resumed control, but the hurt of having a friend end his life never quite went away. And it stayed with me because it was one more secret to keep from a very probing and not very polite press.

The media interest was high not only because of Brad's celebrity but because of the lengths to which Brad had gone to keep his secret, just because he was worried about losing work. His death and his fear while alive focused a lot of attention that had been focused on the Hollywood Establishment. APLA received a call from some of our major donors who wanted to start a Hollywood program for people in the industry who were in Brad's situation. I put together a two-page proposal that was presented to the donors along with the input of folks at the Gay and Lesbian Alliance Against Defamation, and Hollywood Supports was born, providing AIDS-in-the-workplace support for Hollywood.

But I began to get a lot of other calls too. I got an anonymous call from a man who said he was also a star with HIV and needed help. A month later a soap opera star named Dack Rambo, who had been on *Dallas* and who I had never heard of, revealed that he was HIV-positive. I was absolutely incredulous when I began to get mail for him. I found out who his agent was and began forwarding it to him on a regular basis. Later, Rambo actually did come to APLA. We had a meeting, and I gave him any other mail I had for him. But somehow it was perceived that I was Buddy to the Stars. That's why in early November on a Thursday morning Peter Jennings's office from ABC News called me and said that there was someone really big about to come out of the HIV closet. They asked if I could tell them who it was. I said it was news to me. I had the feeling they didn't believe me. Then another call came from another reporter and then another. I called around the building to ask if anyone knew what was going on. It was 10:45 A.M., and no one knew anything.

## IT'S MAGIC TIME

By 11:30 I heard the rumor that the HIV-positive celebrity was Magic Johnson. People were really shocked. My telephone was ringing as if it were having some sort of seizure. Now, much to the disappointment of my father, I had never been a sports enthusiast in any sense of the word. My father had been offered a professional baseball contract at one point in his life and played football while at college at Purdue University. He had tried to introduce me to baseball, but the first time I got hit in the throat with the ball, I said "That's it, brother" and went home. The only sport I ever engaged in was track because you never knew when fast running would come in handy. I dabbled in golf, but my parents were too good and I too intimidated by them to play much. Football seemed just plain ridiculous and basketball, while fun to watch in high school, screaming in support of my home team, was an idea whose time had come and gone. I didn't even know what the name of the team was in L.A., much less who Magic Johnson was and what team he played for.

I couldn't call my father to find out—he was dead. And if he were alive, he probably would have been so disgusted he wouldn't have told me. He would have said something eloquent like, "Well, I'm a goddamned son of a bitch; I can't believe you don't know who Magic Johnson is." It would have been an as- tute observation in all respects but not helpful or timely. My mother, I knew, was a hockey fan. I decided that since the two games are played on fields of seemingly similar proportion, she might know who Magic Johnson is. At least she was loyal enough that she wouldn't laugh at me when I said I didn't know who he was. I could trust her. I cleared a line and called her.

"Hi there!" she said, pleased that I was calling her in the middle of the day.

"Can't really talk, Mom. Listen, I've been getting media calls all morning about someone who is going to admit that he's HIV-positive, and I've found out who it is."

"Who?" she asked, excited to be getting the news firsthand.

"Magic Johnson."

"Wow," she said.

"Do you know who he is?"

"Of course," she said. "Don't you?" Was it my imagination or was she suppressing a chuckle?

"No, I don't. Who is he?"

"He plays basketball for the Lakers." She paused. "That's your team in Los Angeles."

Laughter aside, this is why a good mother is so special. They always come through in a pinch.

"Thanks, I gotta go. I didn't want to admit this to anyone here."

"That's a good thing. Good luck," she said. "Whatever you do, don't mix him up with Michael Jordan."

For the rest of the day I had to act like I knew something about basketball and Magic Johnson. There were plenty of opportunities for me to screw up. Because Los Angeles was home to the Lakers, AIDS Project Los Angeles, as the largest AIDS service organization, was getting hundreds of media calls. ABC, CBS, NBC, ESPN, all the local channels, radio stations I never knew existed, *Sports Illustrated, The Wall Street Journal, The New York Times,* the *Los Angeles Times,* papers in Dallas, Philadelphia, and Chicago all were calling.

So many camera crews were coming to APLA that I realized it would be impossible to interview with each of them. The executive director, the communications director, and the media-relations specialist were all at a conference on the East Coast. I advised the stations and radio folks that we would make a statement at 3 P.M. in our meeting room. By that time I had fully intended to have a press statement, but there were so many calls from print media, I had been unable to get to it. Five minutes before 3 P.M. I walked down to the meeting room. I peeked in and saw dozens of cameras and about a trillion microphones taped to a podium, where in five minutes I would deliver my prepared statement, which I hadn't yet prepared. It all looked so ridiculous. In fact, in hindsight it was all so ridiculous.

I turned around and ducked into an office. There was an electric typewriter there. I put in a sheet of paper and began typing my statement. I type 110 words per minute, and I had only gotten down one-third of the page before I realized that it was simply too late for this. I ripped the sheet out and walked across the hall into the meeting room and up to the podium. A flood of light engulfed me, and I felt like I was staring into the sun. A large number of the staff of the agency gathered in the back of the room to listen. We had never had anything like this before.

"I'm going to make a brief statement, and then I will answer questions," I said, as if I were the president of the United States addressing the press in the briefing room of the White House. I managed to say this without laughing out loud. Then I spoke about how important this was. And as ridiculous as the press frenzy was, the announcement itself was awfully important. One had the sense that most of America had been shaken down to its very foundation with this news. The announcement broke a barrier in the collective consciousness of America, just as the Rock Hudson announcement had. But where Rock Hudson introduced AIDS, a so-called gay disease, to the nation, Magic Johnson stripped away society's naïveté and let us know that straight men get HIV too.

Just as it had been years ago when I did interviews around Rock Hudson's announcement, HIV issues were an education for much of the media in the same way that it was for the general public. Because Magic Johnson was announcing he was HIV-positive, this marked the turning point in the press understanding of the difference between having AIDS and being HIV-infected. So in answering questions, one had to be patient in repeatedly having to make the distinction between the two for people. Many in the general public thought that his announcement meant that he would have only two years to live because that is how long they thought "AIDS patients" lived. It was frustrating but necessary in teaching a public largely uninformed by a largely uninformed media about the biggest health challenge of the century. They aren't entirely to be blamed for their ignorance. You don't learn about these things until someone you know is touched. It is an old adage and well-known fact that people do not change their attitude about AIDS until someone they know is HIV-infected. There was no reason for me to feel self-righteous about this even though ignorant questions could be quite trying. After all, I don't know much about breast cancer. And I wouldn't until someone I know and cared for was threatened by it.

But the other frustration that presented itself was ugly, echoing Brad's death. How did Magic Johnson get AIDS? In cabs, on radio call-in shows, in newspapers, people speculated about his revelation. He stated that he had slept with a great number of women. For so many disappointing people, this was the main question of the entire tragic story. For many, it still is.

The Magic Johnson announcement created a tidal wave, not only of media interest but of funding and interest in HIV. It was a brave thing for him to do, and a smart thing. Eventually someone would have leaked his status in all likelihood unless he took every precaution and lived the way Brad had tried to live. To my mind perhaps the greatest contribution made by his announcement was the effect it seemed to have on young people who idolized a sports hero. It made the mighty vulnerable and breathed life into the dead cliché that this can happen to anybody.

At the end of 1991 then, America was suddenly interested in AIDS in ways that had previously seemed impossible. In November of that year, the month of the announcement, the hotline at AIDS Project Los Angeles received a record number of calls. Teenagers who looked up to Magic Johnson as an idol were stunned and heard the vital message that anyone could be subject to HIV. The slogan that said that "the virus does not discriminate" took on serious meaning for the first time for people. It provided America with one of those milestones, like the JFK assassination.

The press frenzy continued for two days unabated. The announcement was on a Thursday, and on Friday morning I began my day with the Jay Thomas radio show airing at 6 A.M. I woke up early and got to the radio station because I had always had a little crush on Jay Thomas and was happy to be meeting him, even under these circumstances. I arrived in the predawn light to the studio located in the San Fernando Valley and went upstairs to meet Jay, who was just as charming in person as I thought he would be. His cohost chatted with me while we waited to go on the air. They gave me a cup of coffee, which I was sipping from when Jay went on the air saying something like, "Good morning, L.A.! The whole world is talking about the announcement by Magic Johnson that he has HIV, the virus that causes AIDS." This is fine, I'm sipping coffee quietly hoping that the heat from the liquid is going to make my voice sound reasonable on the air. "This morning to help us understand what that means we have Mark Senak from AIDS Project Los Angeles. Mark, why don't we start out by asking you what your HIV status is?" I spit my coffee back into the cup. My eyes go wide, so do those of his cohost.

"Wow, bad question," says Jay, not missing a beat. "Mark, why don't we start out with you telling me why that's a bad question."

Now if I had drunk that coffee instead of spitting it out, I might have been sharp enough to say something gleefully witty like, "Gee, Jay, it isn't a bad question at all if you are wanting a date," but I didn't drink it, and I wasn't all that snappy at 6 A.M. I did recover a fumble nicely, I thought, when I said that taking an HIV test was a very personal decision, and deciding who you are going to tell and when you are going to tell them is likewise very personal. I said I wasn't going to be making that decision on the air. Jay seemed satisfied; I was satisfied. The only problem was that I now had sweat stains down to my hips. The rest of the interview was not memorable. Over the course of that day I had approximately 20 more interviews involving television, radio, and the print media.

The Magic Johnson announcement was certainly one of the milestones of the epidemic. It was the first time there was a wake-up call for heterosexuals, though many would dismiss this in speculation on the mode of transmission for Magic Johnson. It was amazing to me at the time—and now—that people can be so conservative that they don't want specific AIDS information taught to children because it involves sex, yet when the subject is a celebrity with HIV, their morality melts like cold butter on a hot pan of prurience, and sex becomes their number one topic of conversation. For myself, I accept what he said about how he got HIV and don't really care if there is another story because on the whole it would be irrelevant.

The announcement caused a change in awareness and consciousness about the epidemic. HIV/AIDS awareness programs proliferated, and teens were made more aware than ever. But the science didn't really change. For all the well-intentioned efforts and better understanding of virology and the immune system, we were not really any closer to keeping people from dying than we were in 1987. After the thrill of the Magic Johnson moment was gone, the public focus spiraled down. No celebrity announcement would surpass that and nor would any event in HIV history.

The following year, 1992, saw many more such cycles. A sister drug to AZT—ddI—was approved by the FDA, and the press thought this was something new, but it was only sort of the same thing over again. In November 1992 Mike and Allen and I were in Palm Springs for a weekend, so much different from the times before when we had gone there before I lived in California. When I first moved to Los Angeles, Allen looked like he had always looked. What I didn't know directly, I didn't want to know. But Allen had HIV, I just didn't think about it. At that point I would rather not believe such things to be true unless I absolutely had to.

But Allen began discussing his HIV status, and so the denial I had held onto was tossed aside. Still, like Neil and Rick and all the others, I didn't believe that it would actually ever come to Allen getting sick and dying.

When I had visited Mike and Allen one February while Joe was still alive, we went to Palm Springs for a weekend. Allen, who was over six feet tall and powerfully built, spent a lot of time in the pool with me, where we pretended I was Esther Williams and we did "aqua ballet," which really just involved me standing on Allen's shoulders. "Hey, Mike," we'd shout and laugh, thinking we were the cleverest damned guys on the planet. Mike indulged us and took pictures of poor Allen standing in the water smiling while I stood on top of his broad shoulders with my arms held high up as if I were water skiing without a rope. I was amazed that Allen was so strong that he could support me standing up on him like that.

The Allen I came to know by 1992 was no longer that guy. He had become sick and weak and aged 30 years in just two. In November while we were in Palm Springs, he sat nearby while I wrote in my diary, and he was thin and pale and weak with a catheter hanging from his chest. Within a few weeks he became very ill and died in Cedars Sinai before Christmas while Mike attended to his every need. Though I could be in denial about a friend's HIV status as long as it was possible, once serious illness came along I was almost more comfortable with them perhaps because of my early experience with so many deathbed wills. In that way once they were sick I was so resigned to the death of my friends and I think I wasn't entirely there for Mike in the way I would have wanted to be. By the time we had reached our late 30s, men of my generation were like old people in a nursing home. We had seen our contemporaries come and go, and we weren't really sure how long we ourselves would be around. I sat with Mike, I stayed with him at the hospital, but in the end I was helpless to ease the pain I knew he was going to go through. I could only sit back and let it all take its course. I felt like Mike's parent, wanting to spare him the anguish of a situation I had already been through. "Here, I've done this," I wanted to say, "so you shouldn't have to do it too. It isn't fair." I had gotten to say good-bye to Rick a few months before he died. With Allen I said good-bye only hours before he died, and it is the only time with any of my friends that I was aware of the fact that I was doing that—and it is the only time since then. I loved Allen, and when he left, a sweet gentle soul went from us. I remembered a quilt panel I had seen once that said something like, "Why is God picking all of his flowers?"

In December 1992, while Allen was so sick, I flew to Washington for the launching of the Be Here for the Cure Campaign. I made a speech with Pat Christen of the San Francisco AIDS Foundation and the U.S. surgeon general, Antonia Novella, and even though it was a speech about hope, I don't think my heart was really in it.

During the course of the next few years, Magic Johnson would go back to basketball, retire, go back, and retire. No more new drugs made headlines for a while, and even the media seemed to get a little bored. Each time the press called about a new announcement, I got deja vu all over again. Until December 7, 1995, nothing would change. But then, everything would change forever.

# E P I L O G U E : 1 9 9 7

*A cumulative total of 547,742 cases were diagnosed*
*233,475 people were dead of AIDS in America*

---

## GAINING PERSPECTIVE

I often look back at the epidemic and divide it up into eras. The first one I call the Dark Ages, those years between 1981 and 1984 when we knew nothing about what was going on, except that we were scared or at least anyone with any sense was scared. Among those scared people, we saw cowardice and we saw bravery. But I call it the Dark Ages because medical science provided no explanation of what was causing the disease, you couldn't tell if you were infected or not until you got sick, and since we didn't know what caused it or if you were infected, there were no treatments.

The next period of time, 1985 through 1988, I think of as the Years of Enlightenment, because of the dramatic and dizzying speed with which developments suddenly transpired. In 1984 HTLV-III was isolated. In 1985 it became public news that Rock Hudson had been diagnosed, bringing the AIDS epidemic from the background of many people's minds to the forefront of almost everyone's, unfortunately with little resulting education. Soon afterward the HTLV-III antibody test was developed, originally to screen blood for contamination but quickly used by many to screen people instead. It is one of the singular most spectacular events in HIV history. Lastly, in 1986 AZT began to be distributed, fully prescribed by 1987, and at $10,000 per year it was the most expensive prescriptive drug in American history. The exorbitant price was a catalyst for the founding of ACT UP and within two years the cost of AZT was reduced by its manufacturer, Burroughs Wellcome, by 20%.

It was as if the speed of those dizzying events made us all so unsettled that we needed a rest. And so began a long period that I call the Age of Malaise. This isn't quite apt. It isn't that nothing happened, just that the momentum of that second period raised hopes among people connected with the epidemic that in fact there might be progress in seeing an end to this thing. When the virus was isolated in 1984 it prompted then-secretary of Health and Human Services Margaret Heckler to announce that a vaccine would be possible within two years. But the years 1988 to 1995 saw little real development. Doctors did get better at treating the opportunistic infections, and people did live longer than they had before. But they only lived longer to get new and more virulent diseases. In the early years almost everyone either got pneumocystis pneumonia or Kaposi's sarcoma and died. In the later years people like Brad and Neil got MAI or, like my boss while at GMHC, Richard Dunne, got an even rarer disease known as progressive multifocal leukoencephalopathy. Events of significance did occur during this time, one being the passage of the Ryan White CARE Act, dispensing monies to the hardest hit areas of the country for much-needed AIDS supportive services. Likewise, the Americans With Disabilities Act was signed into law in 1990 by George Bush, and stated for the first time in federal legislation that HIV would be considered a disability for purposes of antidiscrimination enforcement. And then, of course, there was the Magic Johnson announcement. But media interest would wain, and AIDS began to take on the character of other social ills that appear chronic, like homelessness or drugs or poverty. In some ways, as a society, we began to embrace our hopelessness that there would ever be a cure or an effective treatment. In 1992 at the international AIDS conference, held in Berlin, one of the plenary speeches was so bleak, I recall sitting in the audience taking notes with tears running down my face. A vaccine, the speaker said, was as elusive as ever, and the truth of the matter was, he explained, that to be truly effective against the global epidemic, any effective treatment would have to be oral and it would have to be cheap. Neither prospect, he said, seemed likely. I think that I had known that already, but I'd never heard anyone confirm it so starkly. There was a great deal of ethnic tension in Berlin that year involving the Turkish population. Almost every day that I was there someone had been fire-bombed or set on fire. It was as if the depressing nature of the conference spilled over and infected the city. It was the worst AIDS conference I ever went to. I came home doubting whether I could go on working in AIDS anymore. I wasn't going to make it. The thought of quitting made me feel as if I was turning my back on every one of my dead friends and on everyone I knew who was diagnosed. Some days at work at AIDS Project Los Angeles, I would volunteer in the food pantry, filling bags of groceries for people and families with AIDS. There is no warmer feeling for me, and yet I would look at their faces with the feeling that I was, sooner or later, going to have to abandon the clients of APLA because AIDS was becoming a chronic social problem, and they would all continue dying, and the quilt would just get bigger and heavier. That was the Age of Malaise, and the speaker's words came home with me and lived with me until December 7, 1995.

That is when the first protease inhibitor, saquinavir, was approved for use by the Food and Drug Administration. Along the years after AZT some sister drugs were introduced, but there were no dramatic changes in the landscape of the epidemic. But protease inhibitors when used in combination with pre-existing drugs were found to be very effective at inhibiting viral replication until the ability of the virus to multiply fell to undetectable levels and the early clinical outcomes were unbelievable. To the credit of the Food and Drug Administration, the drugs were approved in record time, not only for the United States but for the world. When the epidemic began, people often left the United States to go to other nations for treatment, such as Rock Hudson's desperate journey to Paris just before his death to get HPA-23. Many others went to Mexico to get ribavirin. Now, people came to the United States because it has acted so quickly to approve protease inhibitors. What made the change so remarkable was that not only did the drugs appear to work, they were essentially the first thing to come along that really showed an undeniable improvement in quality of life for people with AIDS and HIV. Suddenly we went from an epidemic that was focused on treating people with AIDS and their opportunistic infections to treating people with HIV for the first time. That was the good news. The bad news was and is that the system of health care simply isn't ready for it, particularly given the extremely expensive nature of the drugs and accompanying monitoring tests—$15,000 to $20,000 per year.

All of the public systems for reimbursement are based on people getting poor and disabled. But people with HIV who have not yet developed AIDS or are not yet disabled but are put in the unenviable position of having to get sick in order to qualify for drugs that, if they could get in the first place, they might not get sick. Also, even for those with insurance, many policies have lifetime caps that weren't often reached by a person with AIDS whose life expectancy might be short but that would be hit much more quickly given a $20,000-per-year prescription drug habit. In short, the entire system was really set up for people with AIDS, not HIV, and set up as a system of mortality, not maintenance.

If we don't find a way to deliver the drugs to the large population of people with HIV, there will be a growing class division among people who are the "haves" and the "have nots." While this has always existed, it has never existed on an epidemic scale.

Many of the people who will not receive benefits under the current system are parents. In 1985 there were 233 children orphaned by AIDS in the United States. By 1995 there were over 30,000 such children, and it is estimated that the year 2000 will see over 90,000 children orphaned by AIDS. In a conservative era stressing family values, what about the lives of these families? How can we turn our backs on them? How can this not be a right-to-life issue?

And the problems do not abound merely for the poor. For those who have been out on disability for the past few years, how will we help people go back to work—what about their benefits? Who will hire them? These are tough questions. But they are good questions to have—at last.

Perhaps that is one of the best things about protease inhibitors. While most of the mainstream media jumped once again on the wrong bandwagon and heralded the end or the twilight of the epidemic, in fact, we do not have a cure for AIDS or HIV. But what we did find was a cure for our hopelessness. For the first time in years I don't think about the inevitability of losing my HIV-positive friends. I no longer am frightened of how close I am to them for fear of the terrible pain I will feel upon losing them. That fear is a distant memory.

There is still so much at stake, however. Oliver Sacks relates seven tales of neurological disorder in his book *Anthropologist on Mars.* Each one involves paradox. In one story a man who early in life suffers blindness is given sight back as an adult through a miraculous surgery. It is difficult for any sighted person to imagine a more exciting blessing. But because the man's neural pathways had, over a lifetime, become so attuned to touch, his sight caused him disorientation. He could not tell what an animal was when he saw it, until he touched it—he could not tell which direction a staircase went until he put his foot on it. He became increasingly disoriented and despondent. It is a very similar situation with protease inhibitors. After so long without anything, we have had a miracle. But because our system is so set up for AIDS and not HIV, we stand to see what should be the source of our greatest joy, become the source of our greatest despair.

## LOST AND GONE FOREVER

During 1994 my father's brother died. He had never married and had no children, and under the laws of the state in which he lived, my sister and I inherited part of his estate. It wasn't a lot of money, but it was enough to slap on as a down payment on a small house, which I did. I had been renting a small house in Silver Lake that was located on a lot that had been Disney Studios in the 1920s. The house I rented was reputedly one of the cottages built to house the artists for drawing *Snow White,* one of eight cottages on the lot (one for Snow White, one for every dwarf). I loved living there and it fulfilled many Disney fantasies for me, but I found I was outgrowing it, especially since I had found two baby sheepdogs playing in traffic and accidentally took them in to live with me and my cat, Ginger Pye. (Rupert the Cat died of cancer in 1991.)

Come moving day, however well you plan it, it is always a mess to pack up one's life and tote it somewhere else. Shades of the trip west with Rick crossed my mind, and I found myself sensing some big transition, moving from a lifetime of rental to a state of home ownership. My small car was weighted down with belongings and cat and dogs, and we took off for the new house while the movers I had hired (I had decided I was at an age where you could no longer rely on friends to help you move) began the arduous task of my relocation.

Because there was so much physical work connected with the move, I removed all my jewelry and placed it in a box marked JEWELRY. When we got to the new house, I realized I had left my wallet and checkbook in a drawer at the old house and left the movers to their work while I went and got it. When I came back, thankfully, everything was almost done, and I wrote a check and tipped the guys generously. I began putting everything away, placed Joe's ashes in a suitable spot and sat down and had a little discussion with him on how much he would have liked this and how much I would have appreciated his help if he had been here. There had been more than a few frustrating moments during the week of the move. I had decided to refinish the floors myself, and in the middle of the job, which had been backbreaking and not all that rewarding, I felt so terribly alone, and I resented that Joe was not there to help. After seven years I could still feel the pain of my loss, and I sat in the middle of those half-sanded floors and had a good cry. As the days passed after the move, and I became more settled into the house, it occurred to me that I hadn't come across the box marked JEWELRY. I looked all over for it and couldn't find it. Since I'm frequently absentminded, I didn't panic, but after a week, I took every box that had not yet been unpacked and emptied it into the middle of the den. I searched through everything. The jewelry was gone. There had been nothing of tremendous value in there, except for the two rings from Tiffany's.

This time, I was too hurt to cry. The fact that someone would steal a box of unremarkable jewelry and inadvertently take one of my most treasured mementos of Joe was so confounding to me, I could only sit and blame myself in the most dreadful way. Stupid. It had been the basest stupidity to put the jewelry in a box and label it so obviously, I told myself. Why not just put it in a box marked TAKE ME. It would be my natural tendency to obsess about this. At first I wanted to call the moving company and tell them what I thought had happened. But by the time I had finally determined the rings were missing, three weeks had passed. I had to face it. The rings were gone. And the other thing I had to face was that there was no real blame. I was not to blame, and neither were the movers really. I don't know what motivates people to steal things, but I could only let go of the rings and hope that wherever they went, they brought the same meaning into the lives of their new owners that they brought into my life. They were, after all, only things. Other than photographs, they were really the last things I had left, and certainly the only tangible symbol of the fact that I had been in love with someone and he with me. But the bottom line was they were only things.

Every so often I would still get an aching desire to rub them the way I used to absentmindedly with my thumb, like someone with an amputated limb that still itches. But I found a certain peace about it and even felt good about the way I had handled it. Rather than steep in a pool of anguish and accusation, I just sort of settled down into a Zen attitude about the fact that they were things and that things, like lives, come and go and that I still had that which was most important to me, my sense of good being and my memories of my favorite time of my life.

A year and a half later on the Friday before Thanksgiving in 1996, I was walking across the parking lot outside my office when the strap to my briefcase broke. When I got home that night, I decided to replace the briefcase with my old one. I went to a closet and dug it out and emptied the contents of the broken one. Then I pulled open the compartment of the old brief case where I was going to put my calculator and check book, and there I saw two Tiffany's boxes. I let out a little yelp and pulled them out. I knew that they must be empty. I set them on my desk and slowly opened one up and then the other. There were both of my rings.

What's been lost can be found again. Friends and acquaintances ask me why I haven't settled down with anyone since Joe. I'm not terribly sure of the answer to that. I know that there was no one I had met who seemed to inspire the extreme devotion and love I felt for Joe. And I have come to accept life on those terms.

On a cold and drizzly morning in 1996 I got up early, as is my custom, and lumbered to my front door to get the paper. The sky was predawn gray, and a fine mist was falling. I didn't have my contact lenses in but could see that across the street there was a small stray black dog. He looked like a small Scottie.

"Hey, buddy," I said. "Hey, buddy, what are you doing there all alone? How come you're out in the rain, little guy?" The last thing I need is another dog, being the happy owner of two already.

The dog took notice of me and perked up his head to get a better look. Almost without hesitation, he began to scurry toward me. I could hear his toenails hitting the asphalt pavement. He reached the curb and jumped down and began crossing the street.

I encouraged him—"Come on, buddy!"

He reached my curb and jumped up, and it wasn't until he was half way up my front porch that I could see that he was not a Scottie; he was a skunk. I quickly slammed the front door just as he reached the top step. I opened the trap door set inside my front door and looked down at him. He just stood there, looking at me with very sweet almond-shaped eyes, as if to say "what did you call me all the way over here for if you were just going to slam the door in my face?"

Well, that is what husband hunting in Los Angeles is like. From far away, within the fine mists of distraction, there are a lot of cute puppies out there. But every time I have gotten close to one, skunk city.

Just because it is unexpected does not mean it can't happen. I did meet someone who touched me in such a way that I felt a deep and profound love I didn't know I was capable of anymore. It is nice to know that such a thing is possible again. That feeling broke through all the walls around my heart. Finding the rings didn't give me Joe back, but finding what I had lost was a moving and profound experience. Meeting this man didn't make me married again, but it too has been moving, and my feeling for him is like finding those rings again.

---

The experiences I've had are far different from what they would have been had I always chosen the path of least resistance. It would have been so easy not to play in this game of dodgeball. But what I've encountered out here playing this senseless game is an insight into both the capacity of human warmth and the degree to which we can fail. I would not have otherwise had the benefit of seeing this so clearly. I've seen things I never wanted to see and had to feel things I would have paid good money to avoid. But the fact that I did see and feel them has made me into a different person. I've drawn courage from deep down in myself that I never would have known was there. The epidemic gave me courage where I had none.

Not long ago, a physician with HIV was interviewed on the program *60 Minutes*. He had become infected when he accidentally made a slip of the knife and cut himself while working on a cadaver of an HIV-positive individual. His status has meant incredible heartache, and now he must live with the uncertainty of having a life-threatening condition. But when asked whether he would take back that moment when the knife slipped, he doesn't hesitate; he says no. That is not an uncommon reaction, as bizarre as it may sound. No one wants to get AIDS, but the experience of being faced with the facts of life-threatening illness inevitably causes one to appreciate life in a way that was never fathomed before the illness. That is the way I feel about my experience. I can't say I would have chosen this. If someone came up to me and told me that they could heal any pain I might still feel by erasing the memory of all that I've felt and seen and done, I wouldn't take them up on it. Not for all the money in the world. I wouldn't have chosen this life, but I wouldn't trade it either.

But slogans and quotes don't offer much long-term comfort. For the two years I had with Joe I have had many more to look back and reflect and try to recover from the loss. And like so many I had to do it while suffering more loss, while I watched the tragedy of the epidemic keep unfolding.

In the wildfires that ravage the western part of the United States, there is a wonderful paradox. As devastating as the fires are, and for all of the lives destroyed by them, people and wild animals, the beauty of a forest reduced to charred rubble, there is a rebirth. One type of pine produces a cone that when dropped is only opened by the extreme heat of a fire, so that the seeds can be released. The disaster and the rebirth are thus one and the same. Without the fire, there is no destruction, and without the fire, there is no rebirth.

One thing has kept me going throughout the years of work in the epidemic. Some would project onto the epidemic their own feelings about sex and would say that it was a warning call from the Almighty to mend our sexual ways. On a personal level it has helped me appreciate my humanity. But I need more than that. All those people didn't have to die to teach a moral lesson or to bolster the sagging self-perceptions of people like myself. In the final analysis I have to believe that the AIDS crisis means much more than that. Twenty years ago there was no such thing as AIDS and no such known animal as a retrovirus. Today there is AIDS, and the epidemic has resulted in a scientific understanding of the retrovirus to a degree that would have otherwise never occurred. Moreover, insight into the functions of the immune system grew exponentially as a result of the crisis. It is possible that new protease inhibitor therapies will someday be employed for disease conditions other than AIDS. Research into the genetics of viruses and the engineering of genetics to provide insight into healing might one day result in a cure, not only for AIDS but for other diseases such as cancer. I have to believe that I lost Joe—and that the thousands of others who have suffered their losses have done so—for the benefit of something yet untold and that either HIV is going to have tremendous collateral benefit for people suffering from all sorts of diseases or that it has provided us with the research we will need to fend off some greater viral malady as yet unknown, just as HIV itself was unknown only 20 years ago. This HIV infection is spread only through very prescribed circumstances. But who knows, with the next unknown virus, we may not be so lucky. Maybe the next one could be spread by casual contact. Twenty years ago this might have sounded like science fiction, but then so would have the AIDS epidemic.

In the end I have to accept that the meaning of these deaths, and all of this suffering remains unclear. I don't know that anything I've learned has been worth the price. The notion that all of this has meant something is as hard to hold on to as anything I've experienced in this life. It is a difficult notion to embrace, but I do believe in it. That is what faith is.

---

A news report shows officers who have been involved in an extremely violent shootout with bank robbers in North Hollywood in the spring of 1997. It is an unusual press conference because the officers are talking about what it felt like to be outgunned and how victimized they felt when they were confronted with the superior fire power. It wasn't fair; they were, after all, the good guys. What makes this press conference even more unusual is that the officers talk how close they came to dying themselves. One big guy tells how he arrived at the scene while the bank robbers were still inside, and he tried to clear the streets. "Something told me to look up," he said, "and I saw one of them aiming his AK-47 at me. I ducked behind a van, and then it began to explode with bullets." On the videotape being run as he speaks, he hears bullets hitting civilians, and he begins to cry. A fellow officer comes over and puts his arm around this big strapping guy whose voice has cracked and comforts him while he wipes away tears. Another older veteran describes his feelings while watching the video reliving his near-death experience, and his voice too cracks, and he falters when he talks about what it was like to hear the words over the radio "Officer down." Though painful for them, I think it's a good thing, as exceptional as the news conference may be. They have been through a moment that defined the rest of their lives, and they're dealing with their feelings about it in an open and honest way. There are no guarantees; the next time the officer may not hear the voice telling him to "look up."

I watch, knowing all too well what they're talking about. For those of us who have nearly gotten blown away by this epidemic, not knowing if we were going to die, not knowing what we can do as the bullets hit our civilians—for those of us who have looked up to see a gun aimed at our heads—it has been a long day. I know what these officers are talking about, and I'm glad that for them this brutal experience lasted only for a day. I'm sorry ours has lasted for so many years. I'm sorry that I have had to hear about so many men who are down. Like the officers, I have a lump in my throat, glad to be alive and glad to know that in the final analysis, none of us is so very different from each other. We all face our defining moments, and we don't ever forget them; we just learn how to live with them. Recognizing those moments in one another is what gives us our humanity.

Later that week I go to mass. I find a comfort in the ritual and mystery of the mass, in the faith it demands. There are two moments in the mass that are my favorite. In the first the priest bids us each to give one another the kiss of peace, and we all turn to those around us and shake hands, wave, or kiss. I love the community of that moment, the oneness.

My second favorite time in the mass is a paradox of both the mundane and the mysterious. The entire act of communion is about faith, your faith in what you believe, your faith in the transformation of water and bread to blood and flesh. After communion the priest begins the job of cleaning up. The communion hosts, the body of Christ, have been put into as many chalices as are needed to dispense the hosts to the congregation. Afterward, all leftover hosts are gathered back into one chalice. The other chalices that have been used are wiped of crumbs, which are dusted off into one chalice into which the water is poured. All plates that had held the host are dusted off into the single chalice. In this way no morsel of the precious host is lost. I watch as the priest places the chalice before the attendant who pours in a small amount of water. He then puts the cup on the table, and I smile as I watch him ever so gently dip the ends of his fingers in the water. Every morsel, every crumb of communion host is so very precious that it must be saved and not wasted—even the residue on his fingertips is washed off in the water, which he then drinks. Nothing has been wasted. Not everyone in the congregation understands the entire act of communion, but it is part of the mystery that is their faith. You don't have to understand; you just have to have faith.

I understand this too. In one of my drawers, wrapped in a plastic bag, is a pillow case. It is the one that covered the pillow that Joe carried with him through his last ordeal in the hospital. It is the pillow case upon which his head rested when he died. It had collected much of the oil from his hair, and his sweat from the fear of those loathsome procedures. Ever so rarely I go to the package and unwrap it and hold the case to my nose and gently inhale, and there he is. Smell is such a powerful trigger for the memory. I can hear him and see him and feel the fine touch of his skin and memories flood my mind, images more real than memories, and each of them is a morsel so precious to me. Every memory a morsel. I let them linger in my mind; it all becomes quite real, in some ways more real than it was the first time. During this time I don't have to understand the epidemic or why my friends died or why I am here or what came first, Accident or Providence, or which of them is ruling my life. I just have to breathe in and remember, and then for just a few moments, I can remember the intensity of my love. Like the priest, I don't have the miracle itself, and like the congregation, I don't have to understand it. I just have the mystery of my faith and each precious memory. For a moment I can recall what it is to have poetry by night, grateful that I ever had it at all, while I can still appreciate what is still at my fingertips.